The Book of MACROBIOTICS

D0565628

By the same author

The Book of Dō-In: Exercise for Physical and Spiritual Development
Natural Healing through Macrobiotics
How to See Your Health: The Book of Oriental Diagnosis

The Book of MACROBIOTICS

The Universal Way of Health and Happiness

by MICHIO KUSHI

Japan Publications, Inc.

Published by
JAPAN PUBLICATIONS, INC., Tokyo and New York

Distributors:
UNITED STATES: *Kodansha International/USA,Ltd., through Harper & Row, Publishers, Inc., 10 East 53rd Street, New York, N. Y. 10022.* SOUTH AMERICA: *Harper & Row, Publishers, Inc., International Department.* CANADA: *Fitzhenry & Whiteside Ltd., 195 Allstate Parkway Markham, Ontario L3R 4T8.* MEXICO AND CENTRAL AMERICA: *HARLA S. A. de C. V. Apartado 30–546, Mexico 4, D. F.* BRITISH ISLES: *International Book Distributors Ltd., 66 Wood Lane End, Hemel Hempstead, Herts HP2 4RG.* EUROPEAN CONTINENT: *Fleetbooks, S. A., c/o Feffer and Simons (Nederland) B. V., Rijnkade 170, 1382 GT Weesp, The Netherlands.* AUSTRALIA AND NEW ZEALAND: *Bookwise International, 1 Jeanes Street, Beverley, South Australia 5007.* THE FAR EAST AND JAPAN: *Japan Publications Trading Co., Ltd., 1–2–1, Sarugaku-cho, Chiyoda-ku, Tokyo 101.*

First edition: June 1977
Twelfth printing: April 1985

ISBN 0–87040–381–8
LCCC No. 76–029341

Printed in U.S.A.

Dedication

This book is dedicated to the everlasting dream of mankind, past, present, and future, for health, peace and happiness.

This book is also dedicated to those, known and unknown, who have devoted their lives to inspire many people, ancient and modern, Eastern and Western.

This book is further dedicated to all our ancestors and to all offspring not yet born, as well as to living parents and children,

The offering of this dedication is shared by George and Lima Ohsawa and many world friends, along with my parents, Keizo and Teru Kushi, my wife Aveline, and my children—Lillian, Norio and Candy, Haruo, Yoshio, and Hisao.

When we eat, let us reflect that we have come from food which has come from nature by the order of the infinite universe, and let us be grateful for all that we have been given.

When we meet people, let us see them as brothers and sisters and remember that we have all come from the infinite universe through our parents and ancestors, and let us pray as One with all of humanity for universal love and peace on earth.

When we see the sun and moon, the sky and stars, mountains and rivers, seas and forests, fields and valleys, birds and animals, and all the wonders of nature, let us remember that we have come with them all from the infinite universe. Let us be thankful for our environment on earth, and live in harmony with all that surrounds us.

When we see farms and villages, towns and cities, arts and cultures, societies and civilizations, and all the works of man, let us recall that our creativity has come from the infinite universe, and has passed from generation to generation and spread over the entire earth. Let us be grateful for our birth on this planet with intelligence and wisdom, and let us vow with all to realize endlessly our eternal dream of One Peaceful World through health, freedom, love, and justice.

Having come from, being within, and going towards infinity,

May our endless dream be eternally realized upon this earth,

May our unconditional dedication perpetually serve for the creation of love and peace,

May our heartfelt thankfulness be devoted universally upon everyone, everything and every being.

Preface

In August 1945, World War II ended with miseries of destruction in Europe and Asia. Hundreds of millions of people suffered and died during the long years of this war. Soon after the war ended, other wars began to break out in various areas of the world. Concurrently, with the increasing technological prosperity of modern civilization, the degeneration of humanity began with rapid speed.

During my late teenage years I often visited shrines, praying for the spirits of the dying soldiers, many of whom were my friends, wondering why we had to fight on this earth. In my early twenties, my questioning was extended to various other undesirable human affairs, including sicknesses, disagreement, selfishness and egocentricity, searching for the universal way towards eternal happiness.

I am grateful that I could meet George Ohsawa while I was a World Federalist studying in the graduate school of Tokyo University and Columbia University; the Reverend Dr. Toyohiko Kagawa, a Christian leader; Professor Shigeru Nanbara, Chancellor of Tokyo University; Toyohiko Hori, Professor of Tokyo University; many other seniors in Japan; and Albert Einstein, Thomas Mann, Upton Sinclair, Norman Cousins, Robert Hutchins, and other seniors in the United States. I am also grateful that I could have various work experiences—as dishwasher, bellboy, night watchman, interpreter, retailer, trader, restaurant operator, correspondent. Throughout this period, I continued to study various sciences to be synthesized for the health and happiness of mankind. Oriental philosophy, medicine, and culture needed to be synthesized with modern Western sciences for a comprehensive understanding of human destiny.

In order to bring about a unified world, it is necessary to establish a unifying principle which covers all domains of religion, philosophy, science, and culture, as well as all physical, mental, spiritual, and social phenomena. The universal principle of change, yin and yang, which forms the background of all Oriental societies and ways of thought, should be verified and confirmed by modern research and information.

I began to lecture in New York in 1955. With many friends, I continued to talk about the way of life according to the order of the universe. I have been living day and night with the unchanging dream for the realization of one peaceful world. Especially since 1963, many of my student friends have started to spread the way of life for health, freedom, and happiness, throughout America, Europe, and other parts of the world, coordinating with many international friends.

For the same dream, we have promoted the natural food movement along with the macrobiotic principle, and we have distributed the ideological, cultural ground for one peaceful world, including the introduction of Oriental philosophy, medicine and culture to Western countries, out of gratitude for what Eastern countries have received from the West for the past 100 years.

During these 14 years, nearly 10,000 stores in North America have started to carry natural foods, as well as a few hundred restaurants; and many organic farms have begun. Alternative medicine, including Oriental medicines such as acupuncture, shiatsu massage, palm healing, and proper dietary practice, have been spreading in Western society. Peaceful biological revolution has begun to recover humanity from degeneration towards the reconstruction of the world. Macrobiotics has spread to all continents, covering most major countries.

This book is a simple introduction to the principles of health and happiness through the dietary approach based on the way of life according to the order of the universe, macrobiotics. The contents of this book represent a part of what I have discussed in the past 5,000 lectures and seminars conducted in America and Europe. Although the East West Foundation, *East West Journal*, and other related organizations and friends have issued publications on various topics discussed to date, this book has been specially written at the request of Japan Publications, Inc. Miss Olivia Oredson has edited the contents with the assistance of Miss Janet Lacey. Mr. Peter Harris participated in preparing the drawings. I extend thanks for their collaboration along with the support of my many international friends.

February, 1977
MICHIO KUSHI
Brookline, Massachusetts, U.S.A.

Contents

The Degeneration of Modern Man

Since our galaxy was formed by whirlpool motion in the infinite space of the ocean of the universe, and our solar system began to form within the galaxy, an unknown time has elapsed. While the earth developed to nearly its present condition, more than four billion years have passed. Biological life has existed on this planet for more than three billion years, and our mankind has had its progressive development for probably over 20 million years. Although it is uncertain how the ancestors of our human species were living and adapting to their environment, during our recent development as homo sapiens, especially within the span of recorded history, we have seen more than 20 major civilizations rise and fall.

During these constant vicissitudes, we, mankind, have experienced health and sickness, chaos and stability, war and peace, poverty and prosperity, happiness and unhappiness, as if we have been riding upon waves. Our present civilization and this modern age are not exempt from these fluctuations.

Our modern civilization has been offering material wealth and technological conveniences to the majority of the world's populations, together with ample information and varieties of knowledge. At present, we are seeing the blossoming of such benefits: worldwide distribution of food for everyone's survival; transportation which enables us to be on the opposite sides of the globe within the same day; communication systems through which we can know instantaneously what has happened on other continents; well-organized religious and educational programs; universal control of governmental administration; and an impressive degree of scientific and technological development. It is no longer only a daydream that we may colonize other planets. To the far depths of the ocean, to the far reaches of space, to the far ends of the polar regions—our explorations are penetrating everywhere. From the microscopic world of atoms and pre-atomic particles, to the macroscopic world of galaxies and constellations, our understanding is expanding. It appears that we are approaching the realization of the Golden Age.

However, when we examine our surroundings more carefully, we find that everywhere there is sickness instead of health, chaos instead of stability, war instead of peace, poverty instead of prosperity, unhappiness instead of happiness. The huge expenditures of major governmental and public programs are not being applied for the creative development of human potential, but rather, are being used up simply in defensive measures against various negative factors. These negative aspects of modern civilization are as follows:

1.   Endless Expansion of the Defense System
While we are enjoying world trade and exchange as well as global travel, every nation is constantly manufacturing weapons and strengthening its defense forces to prepare to destroy other nations. The potential power of destruction possessed by modern nations can destroy the entire earth within a few hours.

2. Endless Expansion of Medical Care

At the same time that we are making great advances in medical research and health technology, we see more people suffering with sickness—physical, mental, and spiritual. Many large hospital facilities are fully crowded with patients, and many drugstores on every corner are visited from morning to evening by a constant stream of people.

3. Endless Expansion of the Insurance System

While we believe that our life expectancy has been prolonged and social safety has been almost assured, various insurance systems to meet occasions of sickness, accident, injury, unemployment, fire, theft, loss of personal belongings, damage to property, and death, as well as many other difficulties, are constantly developing. Literally every modern person has two or three insurance policies, on the average. This trend is a manifestation of instability in physical and mental health and social conditions.

4. Endless Expansion of Judicial and Police Systems

While we have been convinced that as modern education prevails, violence, greed, selfishness and crime would decrease, in reality, more and more powerful judicial and police control is required to meet the constant increase of undesirable thought and conduct. It is a growing trend that even within our schools, violence and distrust are becoming widespread.

5. Endless Increase of Family Decomposition

While worldwide communication systems are developing in modern society, understanding among family members is becoming increasingly difficult. Only half a century ago, divorce and separation of married couples was uncommon; but at this time, the majority of marriages—8 out of 10 in the case of the United States—meet with divorce or separation. It would soon become a common universal practice. Furthermore, disagreement between parents and children is widespread throughout modern society, with no effective cure in sight.

6. Endless Disorder in Sexual Behavior

As manifested in the increasing rates of divorce and separation, sexual behavior between man and woman is losing its connection with the natural order. Homosexual, bisexual, and group sexual practices are increasing without end. The relationship between man and woman is the fundamental unit of society, and carries within it the promise for future generations. When it loses its natural order, the future of the human species is at stake.

7. Endless Decline of Traditional Spirit

Religious traditions which have inspired people's consciences for many centuries have declined, and their establishments have lost their attraction for the people. School and other educational institutions which in the past have guided people to social awareness, have lost their influence, and their function has changed to one of merely giving out information and promoting competition. Family and community heritage, which has cultivated a rich and valuable spirit for the following generations, has all but disappeared.

In this worldwide prosperous society, most of modern mankind is full of fear and anxiety, wandering in vain, seeking happiness and fulfillment. What mistake have we made in the process of constructing this modern civilization? What we are confronting is the biological, psychological, and spiritual degeneration of mankind, which may lead either to the gradual extinction of homo sapiens by increasting disorder in our physical and mental conditions—or to instantaneous extinction by world destruction through nuclear warfare. Everyone in the modern world is in the middle of a biological Flood of Noah. Where can we find the Ark to save our lives?

In the ancient, geological, Flood of Noah, salvation was achieved by building the Ark; but in this present biological crisis, salvation lies within our own physical, mental, and spiritual constitutions. We need deep self-reflection to discover what mistakes we are making, and we need a biological revolution so that we may change our own constitutions. This is not accomplished by the work of the government; it is not the mission of the church; and it is not the duty of the school. This is our own personal effort for changing our quality of blood and body fluid, improving every one of the billions of cells in our body and brain, and developing our physical health, mental clarity and spiritual awareness.

This self-revolution to re-establish our biological, psychological, and spiritual constitution begins with two bases:

(1) The understanding of what man is, what life is—our origin, and our future— and as a whole, the understanding of the order of this infinite universe.
(2) The biological, psychological, spiritual, and social application of the order of the universe, commencing with proper dietary practices, according to the environmental conditions.

This revolution is the most peaceful and effective way. Through it, we are able to save ourselves from the vast current of degeneration; we are even able to turn the general trend of modern civilization to a more healthy, constructive direction; and, ultimately, we are able to open the door of the new world, the era of humanity, with health and peace, justice and freedom, toward the unlimited happiness of all mankind.

chapter 1

The Order of the Universe

We all have come from infinity,
We all live within infinity,
We all shall return to infinity,
We are all manifestations of one infinity,
We are all sisters and brothers of
one infinite universe.
Let us love each other,
Let us help each other,
Let us encourage each other,
And let us all together continue to realize
The endless dream of health, love, peace and justice
on this earth.

May, 1976

1. Life Is Vanity

The order of the infinite universe, the eternal principles of change, are nothing but the different names of the living God or the moving infinite universe. When the name of God is used, it is often misunderstood as a static personality, and when the term Infinity is used, it is difficult for many people to comprehend. The Infinity of God is neither a person nor a phenomenon; it is a whole oneness, embracing everything —every being, every phenomenon; and it is the endless universe itself. The universe does not remain in one state, but is changing constantly—continuously transforming, eternally transmuting from the beginningless beginning to the endless end. The infinite universe is a perpetual dynamic change within which countless changes are arising everywhere in every dimension and at all times.

Without knowing the order of the universe, it is worthless to talk about life or truth, and it is senseless to speak of the way of man and of his life. Without understanding the order of the universe, no one can achieve health, freedom, and happiness through his own initiative; no society can achieve order, progress, and harmony; no country can complete her security, prosperity, and development; and no world can establish peace and justice.

Where there is no understanding of the order of the universe, there is no true love, no real truth, and no true happiness. It may appear from time to time that there is love, peace, and happiness among people, but it shall pass away in vain,

---

Though a river streams endlessly, yet the water of the stream is not the same. Foams floating on the stream appear and disappear and do not last long. People and their homes in this world are changing constantly. [Chomei Kamo: 鴨長明: *Hojoki* (方丈記) (*Writings in a Small House*)] — 13th century. Beginning part.)

like morning dew, and it shall vanish like foam on a stream. Needless to say, there were in the past, and there are at present, many teachings of a religious and spiritual nature, many discourses of a scientific and intellectual nature, and plentiful knowledge of a social and cultural nature. Love is taught everywhere, health is discussed everywhere, peace is sought everywhere, and grace and salvation are spoken of everywhere. And yet, far and near around us, there are really very few seekers of the order of the universe and the principle of eternal change. And for this very reason, all religious and spiritual teachings have decayed, all theoretic and aesthetic cultures have declined, and all human races and societies have been unable to escape the miseries of disease and poverty, greed and violence.

We hear, here and there throughout the world, voices of consolation, whispers of encouragement. They are calling now as their ancestors called in the past, "Come to us. Your rest is here." But despite that, there are few teachings that reveal the perpetual order of the infinite universe, and even fewer that demonstrate how to practice it. Unless we know ourselves as a manifestation of the order of the universe, we are unable to realize health and love, peace and freedom.

We may see around us injustice practiced upon naive, innocent and good people. We see sickness suffered by those who appear to be practicing the proper way of life. We see daily, people suffering from hardships which appear unreasonable for them. We ourselves at any time may meet with an unexpected accident, sudden death, or unforeseeable misery. We may consider all these things unfair and unreasonable, but acutally there is nothing excepted from the order of the universe. In our ignorance we are unable to see the cause and effect, the mechanism of the movement of life. Everything and anything happens with a certain order by a definite cause and process. In this infinite universe there is nothing that is injustice, unrighteous and improper, because all things have arisen and shall vanish according to the endless order of the infinite movement of the universe. Therefore unless we know the order of the universe, or the justice of the kingdom of heaven, and how to practice it, all of what we are doing in this life, or on this planet, shall turn into ashes. Life is vanity.[1]

The voice of the gong coming from GIONSHOJA (ancient temple of Buddha) echoes a sound of ephemerality. The color of the flowers on the tree of SHARA-SOJU suggests that the destiny of the prosperous is inevitably to decline. Those who are powerful do not last, and disappear like a dream in the spring night. Those who are violent perish like dust in the wind. (*Tale of the Heike*, Vol. 1, Sec. 1—13th century.)

[1] "Vanity of vanities, saith the Preacher, vanity of vanities; all is vanity. What profit hath a man of all his labour which he taketh under the sun? One generation passeth away, and another generation cometh: but the earth abideth forever. The sun also ariseth, and the sun goeth down, and hasteth to his place where he arose. The wind goeth toward the south, and turneth about unto the north; it whirleth about continually, and the wind returneth again according to his circuits. All the rivers run into the sea; yet the sea is not full; unto the place from whence the rivers come, thither they return again." (Ecclesiastes I: 2–7)

2. The Principle of the Universe

The eternal order of the infinite universe is viewed and understood in two ways, as interpreted by George Ohsawa: the seven universal principles, and the twelve laws of change.[2] These two are supplementing each other in endless manifestations of the changing universe. We see them by our intuitive understanding, and we know them as our common sense. Daily we experience them wherever we are, at any time, and no one can deny them. Everything exists in accordance with them, and all phenomena are changing according to them.

The seven universal principles of the infinite universe are:
1. Everything is a differentiation of one Infinity.
2. Everything changes.
3. All antagonisms are complementary.
4. There is nothing identical.
5. What has a front has a back.
6. The bigger the front, the bigger the back.
7. What has a beginning has an end.

The twelve laws of change of the infinite universe are:
1. One Infinity manifests itself into complementary and antagonistic tendencies, yin and yang, in its endless change.
2. Yin and yang are manifested continuously from the eternal movement of one infinite universe.
3. Yin represents centrifugality. Yang represents centripetality. Yin and yang together produce energy and all phenomena.
4. Yin attracts yang. Yang attracts yin.
5. Yin repels yin. Yang repels yang.
6. Yin and yang combined in varying proportions produce different phenomena. The attraction and repulsion among phenomena is proportional to the difference of the yin and yang forces.
7. All phenomena are ephemeral, constantly changing their constitution of yin and yang forces; yin changes into yang, yang changes into yin.
8. Nothing is solely yin or solely yang. Everything is composed of both tendencies in varying degrees.
9. There is nothing neuter. Either yin or yang is in excess in every occurrence.
10. Large yin attracts small yin. Large yang attracts small yang.
11. Extreme yin produces yang, and extreme yang produces yin.
12. All physical manifestations are yang at the center, and yin at the surface.

The terms yin and yang do not represent certain phenomena, nor are they pronouns of certain things. They are showing relative tendencies compared dynamically and therefore to be understood comprehensively. We experience in our daily life on

---

[2] These universal principles and laws of change were comprehensively outlined by George Ohsawa and his associates, throughout numerous descriptions from ancient times to the modern, expressed by various thinkers. Further simplification has been made by the author and his associates, through their experiences and observations of nature and society for the past thirty years.

this earth, for example: in tendency, yin is more expansion, yang is more contraction. In dimension, yin is more space, yang is more time. In position, yin is more outward, yang is more inward. In direction, yin is more ascending and yang is more descending. In color, purple, blue and green are more yin, while yellow, brown, orange, and red are more yang. In temperature, colder is yinner and hotter is yanger. In weight, lighter, yin; and heavier, yang. In natural influence, water results in yin and fire results in yang.

In atomic structure, electrons and other peripheral particles are more yin, while protons and central particles are more yang. In elements, oxygen, nitrogen, potassium, phosphorous, calcium and others are more yin, while hydrogen, carbon, sodium, arsenic, and others are more yang. In light, darker—yin, and brighter—yang. In physical construction, more surface and peripheral—yin, and more inside and central—yang. In vibration, shorter waves and higher frequency are more yin than longer waves and lower frequency, yang.

In work, more psychological, mental, and spiritual are yinner, and more physical, material and social, yang. In attitude, more gentle, passive, receptive—yin; versus more active, positive, and aggressive—yang. In the biological world, the vegetable kingdom is yinner and the animal kingdom is yanger. In the botanical world, the yinner tendency is more leafy, tall, branched, juicy, and of a tropical origin, while the roots and plants that are shorter, more contracted, less juicy, and of a more cold origin are yanger. In sex, female—yinner, versus male—yanger. In body structures, softer and more expanded organs such as the stomach, intestines, bladder and others are more yin than harder and more compacted organs such as the liver, spleen, kidneys, and others. In nerves, more peripheral—yinner, and more central—yanger. In autonomic nervous function, orthosympathetic is yinner, and parasympathetic is yanger. In taste, spicy, sour, and strong sweet are more yin, while less sweet, salty, and bitter are more yang. In seasonal influence, hot summer gives a yinner influence, while cold winter gives a yanger influence.

As we see everywhere in everything, either in its wholeness or in its parts, every phenomenal manifestation in nature and in this universe can be observed and experienced, compared and understood, as either more yin or more yang, or the antagonistic and complementary forces and tendencies which are harmonizing with each other. The proportion of yin and yang in the state of harmony in everything is changing constantly. Thus, everything eventually turns into its opposite. Hot summer changes into cold winter; youth changes into old age; action changes into rest; the mountain changes into the valley; day changes into night; love changes into hate; the rich change into the poor; civilization rises and falls; life appears and disappears; land changes into ocean; matter changes into energy, space changes into time.

They are the eternal laws governing all phenomena, visible and invisible, individual and group, part and whole, past and future. To know them is to reach the so-called tree of life, to drink the water from the river of life, and to live with the justice of the kingdom of heaven. When we discover and know them, all spiritual and religious thoughts, all scientific and philosophical ideas, all individual and social efforts shall come to their achievement by harmonizing all antagonistic and complemental tendencies. They are the highest understanding mankind has ever had, and they are the native genuine intuitive wisdom in everyone. They are the key to realize all possible dreams. By knowing them, we can turn sickness into health, war into peace, conflicts into harmony, chaos into order, and misery into happiness. They are the invincible eternal constitution of the infinite universe, as well as of all phenomena within it, including our existence and destiny, and all worlds.

Examples of Yin and Yang

General	YIN ▽ * Centrifugal force	YANG △ * Centripetal force
Tendency	Expansion	Contraction
Function	Diffusion	Fusion
	Dispersion	Assimilation
	Separation	Gathering
	Decomposition	Organization
Movement	More inactive and slower	More active and faster
Vibration	Shorter wave and high frequency	Longer wave and low frequency
Direction	Ascent and vertical	Descent and horizontal
Position	More outward and peripheral	More inward and central
Weight	Lighter	Heavier
Temperature	Colder	Hotter
Light	Darker	Brighter
Humidity	More wet	More dry
Density	Thinner	Thicker
Size	Longer	Smaller
Shape	More expansive and fragile	More contractive and harder
Form	Longer	Shorter
Texture	Softer	Harder
Atomic particle	Electron	Proton
Elements	N,O,K,P,Ca, etc.	H,C,Na,As,Mg, etc.
Environment	Vibration . . . Air . . . Water . . . Earth	
Climatic effects	Tropical climate	Colder climate
Biological	More vegetable quality	More animal quality
Sex	Female	Male
Organ structure	More hollow and expansive	More compacted and condensed
Nerves	More peripheral, orthosympathetic	More central, parasympathetic
Attitude	More gentle, negative	More active, positive
Work	More psychological and mental	More physical and social
Dimension	Space	Time

* For convenience, the symbols ▽ for Yin, and △ for Yang are used.

3. In Ancient Times

Everything in the universe is eternally changing, and this change proceeds according to the infinite order of the universe. This order of the universe was discovered, understood and expressed at different times and at varying places throughout human history, forming the universal and common basis for all great religious, spiritual, philosophical, scientific, medical, and social traditions. The way to practice this universal and eternal order in daily life was taught by Fu-Hi, the Yellow Emperor, Lao Tzu, Confucius, Buddha, Nagarjuna, Moses, Jesus, and other great teachers in ancient times, and has been rediscovered, reapplied and taught repeatedly here and there over the past twenty centuries.[3]

From observation of our day-to-day thought and activity, we can see that everything is in motion, or in other words, everything changes: electrons spin around a central nucleus in the atom; the earth rotates on its axis while orbiting the sun; the solar system is revolving around the galaxy; and galaxies are moving away from each other with enormous velocity, as the universe continues to expand. Within this unceasing movement, however, an order or pattern is discernible. Opposites attract each other to achieve harmony, the similar repel each other to avoid disharmony. One tendency changes into its opposite which shall return to the previous state. During the day we stand up and are active, while at night we lie down and rest. We repeat this pattern. Being human life, as a single fertilized cell we grow into an embryo, then follow the processes of birth, growth, maturity, and death; then new life repeats the same pattern. These cycles occur everywhere throughout nature.

In *Genesis*, Chapter One, we read, "In the beginning, God created the heaven and the earth." This reveals that One Infinity polarized itself into two complementary and antagonistic forces of yin and yang. *Genesis* then continues the subsequent manifestations or transformations resulting from this polarization, through the stages of vibration (light and darkness), preatomic particles (the firmament, or ionosphere, above the earth), the world of elements (dry land and water), the vegetable kingdom (grass and herbs yielding seed), and the animal kingdom (creatures in the water, on the earth, and in the air), reaching finally humanity, as represented by Adam and Eve, male and female. This entire process of creation took seven days, that is, seven stages of development in the changing universe.

Observing the genesis of the universe and thinking from where we have come, we see that our humanity is the terminus of a huge spiral of life arising in the ocean of One Infinity. The animal kingdom, within which mankind is the last appearance, is within the world of the vegetable kingdom, on which it depends either directly or indirectly for its life and sustenance. There is no clear borderline between these two

---

[3] From thousands of years ago up to the modern age, oriental people have been using yin and yang in expression of their ideas in words and conversation. For example, YIN-SEI (陰性) and YO-SEI (陽性) refer to the nature of people, things and atmosphere. YIN-SEI means yin nature— gentler, slower, dark and humid, and sometimes depressive. YO-SEI, the nature of yang, represents the active, positive, bright and gay, and sometimes aggressive. Then there are the terms YIN-KI (陰気) and YO-KI (陽気): The yin nature of vibration, energy and atmospheric influences is called YIN-KI, while the yang influences are called YO-KI. YIN-KYOKU (陰極), YO-KYOKU (陽極) are used very widely even in modern sciences such as the study of electricity and magnetism. YIN-KYOKU represents the minus pole and YO-KYOKU the plus pole. YIN-DENSHI (陰電子) and YO-DENSHI (陽電子): in modern atomic physics, Far Eastern people call the electron YIN-DENSHI—yin electric particle, and the proton YO-DENSHI— the yang particle. The sun is called TAI-YO (太陽), the Great Yang, and the moon is called TAI-IN (太陰), the Great Yin. Accordingly, China and Japan developed TAI-YO-REKI (太陽暦), the solar calendar, and TAI-YIN-REKI (太陰暦), the lunar calendar. In daily conversation, they use also many expressions such as YIN-U (陰雨)—damp, humid rain; and YO-KO (陽光)—bright happy sunshine.

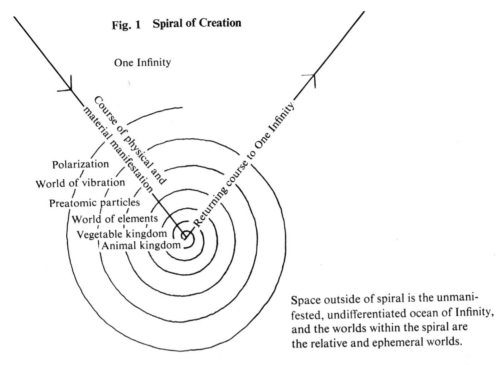

Fig. 1 Spiral of Creation

One Infinity

Course of physical and material manifestation

Returning course to One Infinity

Polarization
World of vibration
Preatomic particles
World of elements
Vegetable kingdom
Animal kingdom

Space outside of spiral is the unmanifested, undifferentiated ocean of Infinity, and the worlds within the spiral are the relative and ephemeral worlds.

worlds, since the vegetable kingdom is continuously transforming itself or changing into the animal kingdom. Thus, one continuing orbit of the spiral leads to the next one within it. Further, the world of vegetables appears originally from the world of elements: soil, water, and air, which is continuously transforming itself into vegetable life. The movement of atoms of the world of elements arises from the manifold spirallic motion of preatomic particles such as electrons and protons which further originate from the waving vibrations of energy. The movement of energy or vibration ultimately appears from two polar tendencies, antagonistic and complementary, or yin and yang, which are the primary manifestations of One Infinity, or the ultimate origin of all phenomena.

Simply speaking, One Infinity differentiates into yin and yang, which begin a spirallic inward process of physical and material manifestation through the continuously transforming worlds of vibration or energy, preatomic particles, elements, vegetable life, and animal life, of which man is the last result. Upon becoming human, we then start to return to One Infinity through an expanding spiral of decomposition and spiritualization, melting personal and individual identities.

In ancient China, this same understanding was revealed by Fu-Hi, (伏儀) (approximately 2500 B.C.), the legendary sage who interpreted the endless change of all phenomena into the eight trigrams. Fu-Hi and his successors used the term TAI-KYOKU (太極), or "ultimate extremity,"[4] to express One Infinity, which polarizes into TAI-IN (太陰), or Great Yin, and TAI-YO (太陽), or Great Yang; these two

---

[4] TAI-KYOKU (太極), ultimate extremity, has also the meaning of MU-KYOKU (無極), which means "non-polarization" or "non-extremity." The One Infinity is expressed by TAI-KYOKU and at the same time by MU-KYOKU.

were symbolized by a divided line (– –) and an undivided line (–) respectively. From this initial polarization, they saw that yin and yang again divide into two, resulting in four; and further, these four again divide, resulting in eight possible combinations or stages of change. This was symbolized as eight sets of three divided and undivided, or yin and yang lines, which are creating the trigrams.

Fig. 2

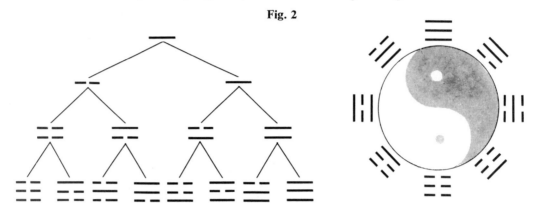

Chart at left shows Tai-Kyoku or Mu-Kyoku differentiate into Great Yin and Great Yang. Great Yin further differentiates into Greater Yin and Lesser Yin; Great Yang further differentiates into Greater Yang, Lesser Yang. Each of them further differentiates into two forming altogether eight variations of phenomena. From left to right, each symbol represents: Earth, Mountain, Water, Wind, Thunder, Fire, Swamp, Heaven. They also represent direction, character, human relations, and various other natural and social, physical and mental manifestations. The drawing at right shows their eternal cycle between yin and yang, manifesting into these eight stages. This chart is used on the universal scale for direction, season, calendars, and other natural and social cycles.

The teaching of Fu-Hi was further developed by many philosophers and thinkers in ancient China, and later became the basis for the 64 hexagrams of the *I-Ching* (易経) or *Book of Changes*. Both Confucius (孔子), (551–479 B.C.) and Lao Tzu (老子) (604–531 B.C.) studied these laws of change and based their teachings on the underlying principle of yin and yang. The work of Confucius includes the *Book of Comments on the I Ching* and Confucianism calls the order of the universe by the term Ten-Mei (天命), the Heavenly Order. On the *Tao Teh Ching*, (道徳経) Lao Tzu wrote of the process of eternal creation:

> "Tao produces One,
> One produces Two,
> Two produce Three,
> Three produce all phenomena.
> All phenomena carry the Yin on their backs
>   and the Yang in their embrace,
> Deriving their vital harmony from the dynamic
>   balance of the two vital forces."

Out of their understanding of the order of the universe, yin and yang, there sprang so-called Confucianism and Taoism, which have widely influenced the way of life in Far Eastern countries for more than twenty centuries.[5]

Also, in the ancient Indian philosophy of Vedanta, which is the origin of Hinduism and Buddhism, and other teachings, we find the principle of dualistic monism expressed in the image of Brahman, or God, differentiating into male (Shiva) and female (Shakti). This universal principle is also expressed in Japanese Shintoism in the *Kojiki* (古事記) (A.D. 712), or *Book of Ancient Events*, and in the *Nihon-Shoki* (日本書紀) (A.D. 720), the book of Japanese history, which were composed from ancient records, legend and mythologies. In these versions on the creation of the universe, One Infinity, named in the image of God, AME-NO-MINAKANUSHI-NO-KAMI[6] (天御中主神), Heavenly Central God, appears in the beginning and TAKAMI-MUSUBI (高皇産霊) and KAMI-MUSUBI (神皇産霊) or the Gods of Centrifugality and Centripetality, manifested thereafter. From these, all phenomena of the entire universe arose in the images of numerous gods and spirits, comprehensively so-called YAOYOROZU-NO-KAMIGAMI, eight million gods. We see the same understanding of the universal principle further in the mythology of the ancient Sumerians in the Mideast and the traditions of the Celts in northern Europe, as well as the original understanding of the universe in Zoroastrianism and here and there in ancient legend in the Yucatan peninsula and northern South America. Greek and Roman mythologies as well as Scandinavian mythologies are not excepted from this understanding in its principles of creation of the universe and life.

The teaching of Jesus[7] was based on the same underlying principle called yin and yang in the Orient. In the *Gospel According to Thomas*, discovered in about 1945 in the Coptic version in the region of the Upper Nile, when his disciples asked,

---

[5] Oriental cultures are all based upon the understanding and application of the order of yin and yang. The way to harmonize yin and yang by using flowers and plants is called the art of flower arrangement, IKEBANA (生花・華道). The way to harmonize them in the manner of serving tea is called Tea Ceremony or SA-DO (茶道). In brush writing, it is called the art of calligraphy—SHO-DO (書道). In martial arts, BU-DO (武道), in all areas such as the art of swordsmanship—KEN-DO (剣道); the art of physical adaptation to the opponent, JU-DO (柔道); and the art of harmonizing *ki*—AIKI-DO (合気道) (KI means physical and mental energy.); the art of archery—the art of unification between the self and the target—KYU-DO (弓道); etc. the word Do is the same as TAO, which realizes the order of the universe in thought and action. Do or TAO is the universal expression of unifying ourselves to the infinite order of the universe such as SHIN-TO (SHIN-DO) (神道), Shintoism; BUTSU-DO (仏道), Buddhism; and SEN-DO (仙道), the way to become free man. Oriental medicine is also called I-DO (医道), to harmonize our life with the environment. The word Do is also written in Japan as MICHI.

[6] KAMI (神) represents the invisible harmony of yin and yang, and when they are manifested into a person he is called MIKOTO (尊・命). In ancient mythological history, both terms are frequently appearing.

[7] The thought of Jesus appears traditionally from Judaism, especially from the teachings of the Essenes which were partly influenced by Pythagorean thought in ancient Greece. However, they are found to be nearest to the thoughts of the ancient Far East. Most of the healing methods performed by Jesus and his disciples are seen also in the ancient Far East. For example, the art of healing by the laying on of hands was widely and commonly practiced in ancient Japan and was known as TANASUE-NO-MICHI (手末の道), the Tao of Palm Healing.

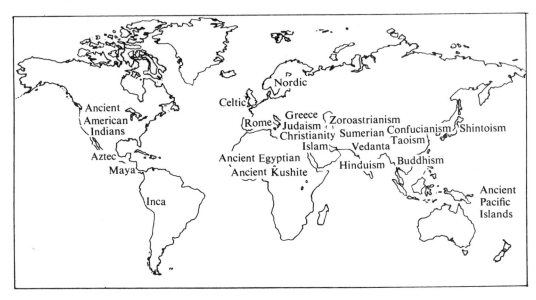

All examples of the above ancient cultures, religions, mythologies, and cosmologies, share dualistic monism which differentiates into two from One Infinity as antagonistic, complementary forces which are the source of the creation of all phenomena.

Fig. 3

"When will the Kingdom come?" Jesus replied that it is nothing else than this infinite universe, saying, "It will not come by expectation; they will not say, 'See, here,' or: 'See, there.' But the Kingdom of the Father is spread upon the earth and men do not see it."[8]

And he further explains, "If they ask you 'what is the sign of your Father in you?', say to them: 'It is a movement and a rest.' "[9]

And he says to his disciples, on how to enter and live within this infinite universe, "When you make the two one, and when you make the inner as the outer and the outer as the inner and the above as the below, and when you make the male and female into a single one, so that the male will not be male and the female not be female, when you make an eye in the place of an eye, and a hand in the place of a hand, and a foot in the place of a foot, and an image in the place of an image, then shall you enter the Kingdom."[10]

Jesus meant, in our terminology, that when his disciples could change yin into yang and yang into yin, and achieve harmony through the unification of both, then they could enter and live in health, freedom and happiness.

The universal principle of yin and yang is the intuitive common understanding which is symbolized respectively in Judaism, Taoism, Shintoism, Buddhism, Christianity, Zoroastrianism, and many others. Together with those religious adaptations, we are able to see the application of the same understanding in various astronomical

---

[8] (Log. 113): Refer to Luke XVII, 20–21; Mt. XXIV, 23; Jn. I, 26.

[9] (Log. 50): Refer to Lk. XVI, 8; Jn. XII, 36; Eph. V, 8; I Thess. V, 5; Jn. VI, 57; Rom. IX, 26.

[10] (Log. 22): Refer to Mt. XVIII, 1–3; (Mk. IX, 36; Lk. IX, 47–48); Mt. XIX, 13–15=Mk. X, 13–15=Lk. XVIII, 15–17; Gal. III, 28; Eph. II, 14–16.

and public constructions as well as in many arts, crafts and other remains from the time of the megalithic age among ancient people throughout the world, until comparatively recent periods when modern civilization spread over the world since about the sixteenth century.

Fig. 4 Religious Symbols

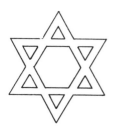
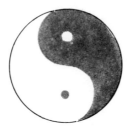
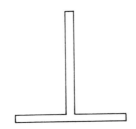
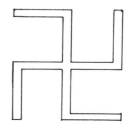

Symbol of Judaism
Harmony between yin and yang, a symbol of Infinity, God Almighty.

Symbol of Taoism
Yin and yang rotate and alternate. The center of the yin half has a yang nucleus, the center of the yang half has a yin nucleus.

Symbol of Shintoism
Harmony between vertical line, HIMO-ROGI (Divine Tree), and horizontal line, IWASAKA (Earth or Ground).

Symbol of Buddhism
Yin vertical, yang horizontal, combine together and rotate, representing universal reincarnation.

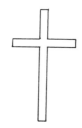
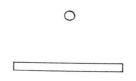
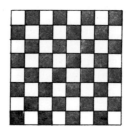

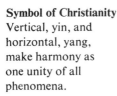

Symbol of Christianity
Vertical, yin, and horizontal, yang, make harmony as one unity of all phenomena.

Symbol of Zoroastrianism
Yang, condensed dot, and yin, extended line, always together, showing universal antagonism and complementality.

Zoroastrian Chart of the Universe
Chart of the Universe: 32 yin white squares, 32 yang black squares, compose 64 appearances of universal phenomena confirming also the 64 hexagrams of ancient China.

4. In the Modern Age

Within relatively recent times, the universal principle of yin and yang has also been observed and applied, directly or indirectly, by many great philosophers and thinkers. For example, among them, Georg Wilhelm Friedrich Hegel (1770–1831), in his interpretation of dialectic development, postulated that human affairs develop in a spirallic form from a phase of unity, which he termed *thesis*, through a period of disunity, or *antithesis*, and on to a higher plane of reintegration, or *synthesis*. Hegel's principle of dialectics was, of course, later studied by Karl Marx, Friedrich Engels, and their associates, and formed the basis of their philosophical speculations in the area of politics, economics and science. Albert Einstein (1879–1955), among many other scientific thinkers of the twentieth century, sensed the complementary antagonism between the visible world of matter and the invisible world of vibration, or energy, and, based on this insight, formulated his universal principle of relativity, in which he stated that energy is constantly changing into matter and matter is continuously becoming energy.

Arnold Toynbee (1889–1975) based his study of history on the alternating movement of yin and yang, which he expressed as *challenge and response*. In one of the early chapters of his multi-volume *Study of History*, he describes, "Of the various symbols in which different observers in different societies have expressed the alternation between a static condition and a dynamic activity in the rhythm of the Universe, Yin and Yang are the most apt, because they convey the measure of the rhythm directly and not through some metaphor derived from psychology or mechanics or mathematics. We will therefore use these Sinic symbols in this study henceforward."[11]

In the past years of the modern time, the relative movement between yin and yang, antagonistic and complementary forces and tendencies, has been partially noticed and applied to many varying domains. The world of electricity as well as the field of magnetism, involves a flow of current and charge between plus (+) and minus (−) poles, yang and yin. The balance of blood is maintained between alkalinity and acidity as well as between red blood cells and white blood cells. Autonomic nerve reactions covering the extensive area of automatic motion throughout the human body respond in the complemental relation between orthosympathetic and parasympathetic nerve actions. Chemical compositions, including DNA and many others, are composed between alternating yin and yang groups of elements. All physical phenomena are conditioned with the antagonistic relation between time and space, mass and energy, and many other relative factors.

This eternal and universal principle of yin and yang has been comprehensively interpreted in the past fifty years, derived from the traditional view of oriental medicine by George Ohsawa (Yukikazu Sakurazawa), (桜沢如一), (1892–1966) and his associates. During his lifetime he successfully reviewed almost the entire scope of the order of the universe and could apply it in pathological treatment through the adjustment of dietary practice and the way of life in general. This application has further been developed towards the understanding of all biological, psychological, and spiritual phenomena as well as natural and social movements, to the extent that the destiny of entire mankind becomes foreseeable. The biological and psychological application in the way of life is called *macrobiotics* in general terminology, derived from the Greek term "macro" for large or great, and "bios" for life. Macrobiotics is the way of life according to the largest possible view, the infinite order of the universe, and it has meant the way of longevity and rejuvenation, as Joseph Need-

---

[11] Arnold Toynbee, *A Study of History*, First Abridged One-Volume Edition, Oxford University Press, 1972, P. 89.

ham (1900–) described in his book *Science and Civilization of China* (Vol. 5, Part 2), as the ancient art of health. The practice of macrobiotics is the understanding and practical application of this of order to our lifestyle, including the selection, preparation, and manner of eating of our daily food, as well as the orientation of consciousness.[12, 13]

5. Spiral: The Universal Pattern

Observing the movement of antagonistic and complementary forces, yin and yang, in the order of the universe, through time and space, we discover that the pattern of their motion is everywhere spirallic as we view from the front, and helical when we view from the side. About 80% of the galaxies, including our Milky Way, are moving in this universal form of the spiral, as well as the currents of wind and ocean upon the earth, the growth and development of plants, the construction of shells found on the beach, the flow of water down the drain, in the whorls of our fingertips, the helical structure of DNA, the construction of our ears, and the spiral pattern of hair growth on our heads.

Fig. 5 Examples of Natural Spirals

Some of them are beautifully formed logarithmically.

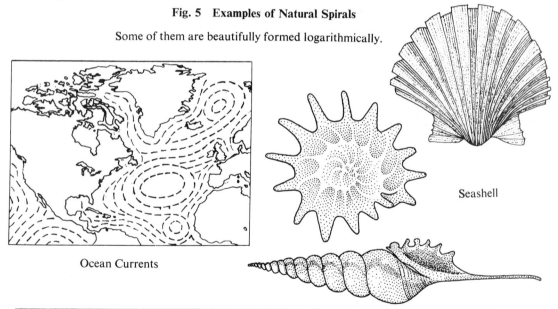

Ocean Currents

Seashell

---

[12] George Ohsawa is well known in Western countries as well through his educational activity and writings. For example, his books include *Zen Macrobiotics, The Book of Judgement, The Macrobiotic Guidebook for Living*, and others.

[13] In oriental countries there have been many other outstanding thinkers who advocated the spirit and practice of the macrobiotic way of life. Among them are, in Japan, Ekiken Kaibara (17th century) (貝原益軒), Shyoeki Ando (18th century) (安藤昌益), Sontoku Ninomiya (18th–19th century) (二宮尊徳), Kenzo Futaki (19th century) (二木謙三) and Sagen Ishizuka (19th–early 20th century) (石塚左玄), who influenced George Ohsawa. Many religious and spiritual people as well as ethical traditional people have also practiced the macrobiotic way of life.

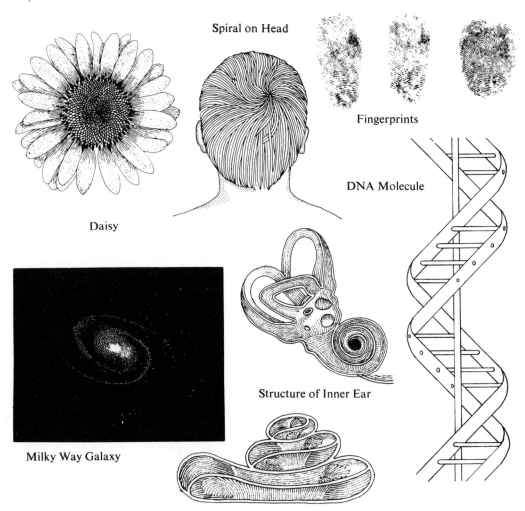

Spiral on Head

Fingerprints

DNA Molecule

Daisy

Structure of Inner Ear

Milky Way Galaxy

Spirals are initially created by a yang centripetal force from the periphery to the center, moving towards physicalization and materialization, and upon reaching their most contracted state this centripetal force turns to its opposite, a yin centrifugal force, expanding from the center back to the periphery, taking a course of decomposition and dematerialization. The periphery, being more expanded, is the more yin region of the spiral, whereas the center, being more condensed, is the more yang region. The ultimate periphery is the infinite space of the universe, the greatest yin, and the ultimate state of condensation is infinitesimal matter, the greatest yang.

When modern science examines electrons and protons in detail, it sees that they are not discrete particles but are regions within the spirallic field of moving energy known as the atom, where the condensation of energy is particularly dense or highly charged. In the case of the proton, this condensed energy is positively charged, centrally located, and therefore yang. In the case of the electron this spirallic cloud of condensed energy is negatively charged and located at the periphery, and therefore yin. However, electrons are moving at a much greater speed than protons, and in this sense their activities are more yang in comparison with the activities of pro-

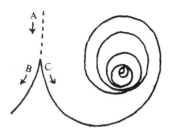

Fig. 6

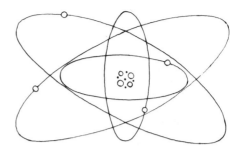

Formation of Preatomic Particles
A. Photon—energy—transforms into preatomic particles. B is the course to produce a proton, C is producing an electron with spirallic motion.

Model of Atomic Structure
Beryllium atom.

tons. So, even though a yang proton is much greater in size than a yin electron, a dynamic balance is achieved through the electron's rapid, yang motion.

The spirallic construction of the universe has left many traces within the human form. In fact, the basic form of bodies is spirallic, though this form can be more clearly seen in the form of the human embryo. The two main complementary-antagonistic spirals in our bodies function through the nervous and digestive systems. While in the womb, the digestive system is originally more yang, being in a central or inward position, while the nervous system, being at the periphery, is more yin. Among the nutritional elements which nourish the embryo through the mother's placenta with her blood, the more yin factors such as proteins are more attracted to the yang digestive system, and in consequence this system eventually becomes more yin, i.e., soft and expanded. In a similar manner, more yang minerals like calcium are attracted more to the peripheral, yin nervous system, which eventually becomes more yang (i.e., hard and compacted), forming the spine.

Fig. 7 Spirallic Development, Embryo to Adult

Beginning Period of Embryo

Fully-Grown Adult

Early Stage of Embryonic Development

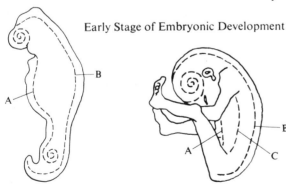

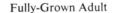

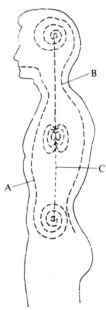

In each of the three drawings, A—the inner system—represents the digestive and respiratory systems. B—the peripheral system—represents the nervous system. C—the middle system—represents the circulatory and excretory systems, which result from the interaction between systems A and B.

Fig. 8   Spirals Seen in the Arm

Each logarithmic orbit of the spiral developed
later as a section of the arm. The tip of the
fingers are the most inner part of the spiral.

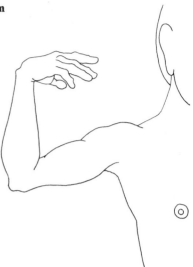

The formation of the arms and legs is also
spirallic. Consider their curled position during
the period of embryonic development as well as
in a new-born baby. The arms and legs are each
composed of seven-orbital logarithmic spirals,
which is the universal form of any complete
spiral within the universe. In the arm, for example, count the root of the arm—which is the
region of the collarbone and shoulder-blade—
as the first orbit; the region from the shoulder
to the elbow as the second; the elbow to the wrist as the third; the area from the
wrist to the knuckles as the fourth; and the three joints of the fingers respectively as
the fifth, sixth and seventh orbits. Also, the distance from the shoulder to the elbow
is about one half the distance from the shoulder to the tips of the fingers; the distance from the elbow to the wrist is about half the distance from the elbows to the
tips of the fingers; the distance between the wrist and knuckles is about half that of
the wrist to the tips of the fingers; the distance between the knuckles to the first joint
of the fingers is half that between the knuckles and the tips of the fingers; and the
distance between the first and second joints of the fingers is about one-half that between the first joint and the fingertips.

From here to eternity, from there to the endless space, everywhere at any time,
logarithmic spirals in all dimensions appear and disappear in the boundless ocean
of the universe. This world of vicissitude governed by two antagonistic and complementary forces, yin and yang, is the relative world, sensed, perceived and experienced by everyone in everyday life. From a tiny flower in the field to large movements of the entire universe, from a shadow of a smile on our face to the huge scale
of natural catastrophe, everything, every being and every phenomenon is spirallically
governed between expansion and contraction, in the relation of front and back, and
in the balance between the beginning and the end.

6. The Spiral of Life

Within the infinite ocean of the universe, a spiral of life has arisen in the seven-
orbital stage of inward movement: First stage, Infinity, the primary source and origin of all phenomena: Taikyoku, Brahman, God, or Oneness. Second stage, polarization, the appearance of yin and yang, centrifugality and centripetality, space and
time, the source of all antagonisms and complementality, the origin of all relative
worlds. Third stage, energy and vibration, manifesting throughout the phenomena

of the world, as the primary state before and after physical and material appearances. Fourth stage, preatomic manifestation appearing in a form of numerous particles which are condensed parts of the spirallic motion of energy. Fifth stage, the world of elements, formed by the spirallic gathering of many preatomic particles manifesting into atomic structure. Their molecules also appear in the states of solid, liquid, gas and plasma, in the physical state; and soil, water, and air in nature. Sixth stage, the world of vegetables, organic manifestations of a part of the world of elements, charged electromagnetically, growing and decaying between expanding and contracting forces upon the surface of the earth. Seventh stage, the animal world which has transformed out of the vegetable world as more highly charged and activated, therefore independent life phenomenon. As its latest development, our mankind has evolved as the most intensively organized active species, both physically and mentally.

The universal process of this centripetal spiral of life reached the center with the creation of man and other highly evolved animal species. The inward course of physicalization in this spiral of life, however, starts to turn at its center to the reverse course, returning again towards the preceding manifestations and ultimately merging into One Infinity, the origin of all. (Refer to the following diagram.)

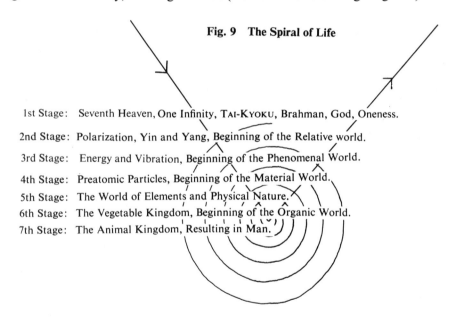

Fig. 9   The Spiral of Life

1st Stage: Seventh Heaven, One Infinity, TAI-KYOKU, Brahman, God, Oneness.

2nd Stage: Polarization, Yin and Yang, Beginning of the Relative world.

3rd Stage: Energy and Vibration, Beginning of the Phenomenal World.

4th Stage: Preatomic Particles, Beginning of the Material World.

5th Stage: The World of Elements and Physical Nature.

6th Stage: The Vegetable Kingdom, Beginning of the Organic World.

7th Stage: The Animal Kingdom, Resulting in Man.

In the process of the emergence of human life, energies, vibrations manifested in the elemental form, organic chemical compounds, absorbed and arranged in the form of vegetables, are taken in the last process of physicalization in the course of millions of billions of years, which began from One Infinity. That is the process of eating, digestion and absorption, through our digestive vessels. The stream of blood changes into the formation of body cells, and the reproductive cells, including ovum and sperm. The formation of the ovum is a result of inward spirallic motion of follicles in the ovaries, yang, while the formation of sperm is the result of differentiation of reproductive cells, yin, both of which therefore attract and fuse with each other to create the beginning of new life. During the embryonic period of approximately 280 days, four major stages are logarithmically taking place in the mother's uterus. The first process is fertilization and implantation, over a period of about seven days. Second, the formation of the major systems takes place, over a period of about 21 days. Third, the major organs and glands become formed along the systems, taking about 63 days. The fourth period of approximately 189 days sees the formation of appendages and continuous development, up to the time of birth.

Fig. 10   The Formation of Sperm and Ovum

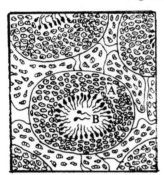

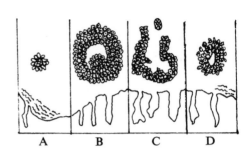

Cross-Section of Testes

A: Immature sperm cells
B: Mature sperm cells

Ovarian Changes with the Production of Ovum

A: Immature follicle and ending of menstruation
B: Maturing follicle
C: Ovulation
D: Degenerating corpus luteum and beginning of menstruation

During this embryonic period, our growth and development is made by autonomic, mechanical operations which we may call the primary and basic judgment of our life. Upon birth and to the end of our human life, this primary judgment continues to function through all parts of our body, such as unconscious nerve reactions, digestive and respiratory functions and circulatory and excretory activities, in various ways. However, soon after our birth we begin to develop sensory consciousness or judgment to deal with various kinds of environments: sense of touch for the solid environment, sense of taste for the liquid environment, sense of smell for the gaseous environment, sense of hearing for the vibrational environment, and sense of sight for the world of light. The sensory experience further involves various physical desires such as hunger and appetite, pain and comfort, heat and cold, and many others.

In the third stage, on the basis of sensory experiences, we continue to develop our emotional, sentimental judgment or consciousness, which deals with the feeling and distinction of beauty and ugliness, love and hate, joy and sadness, like and dislike, emotional attachment and detachment, sentimental agreement and disagreement. This is the world of *Romeo and Juliet*, the *Tale of Genji*, *Don Quixote*, and *War and Peace:*

Through the repeated experience of sensory and sentimental rise and fall, we grow and develop our judgment and consciousness to the fourth, intellectual level: assumption and speculation, conceptualization and organization, analysis and synthesis, evaluation and definition—all other similar mental activities, working more objectively. In this level, logical concepts are formed, reasoning images are structured, organized systems are conceived and comparative values are defined. This is the world of modern science and technology, as well as social administration.

Our consciousness further expands towards the relation among people, societies, and worlds. From individual human relations we further develop to understand and balance family relations; from family relations to community relations; from community relations to relations among humanity and other species. This level of consciousness may be called Social Judgment. The problems of ethics and morals, harmony and peace, balance in power and in economy are among many other concerns in this level. This level controls a personal life from the view of society and a national policy from the view of the benefit of the world.

Our consciousness further grows through numerous successes and failures in the experience of all preceding levels of judgment to the level of ideological thought —What is life? From where have we come? To where shall we go? What is the purpose of this life? Who am I? We start to reflect upon the meaning of our life, seek the secret of the universe, and want to have revealed the eternal truth. This sixth level of ideological consciousness is a door to the last level of consciousness. All traditional religions, doctrines, and teachings of the way of life begin at this ideological level.

Through the constant search for universal truth, the meaning of life, the origin and future of life, we finally reach the universal consciousness, which may be called Supreme Judgment. This level is our understanding of the order of the universe and the attainment of universal love and absolute freedom. Reaching this universal consciousness and living with it as a manifestation of the order of the universe, is the so-called entering into *satori*, nirvana, or the state of Buddha. This consciousness does not conflict with any phenomenon, embracing all contradictions in this ephemeral world, understanding the paradoxical constitution of the entire universe and beginning to exercise our real freedom. At that time, we all become our own master with nothing against us and live with the spirit of endless gratitude and love—One Grain, Ten Thousand Grains—and pray to realize eternally our endless dream.

However, the majority of modern people limit themselves only to either the second, sensory or third, sentimental and emotional world, seeking ephemeral value in the changing world. Few among them enter into the fourth intellectual level and further fewer grow to the fifth, social and sixth, ideological levels of consciousness. Very few, from time to time every several hundred years, appear among the people, who are able to attain and play with universal consciousness, Supreme Judgment. It is, however, not impossible for everyone when he knows the order of the universe and its endless mechanism of change, yin and yang, together with how to practice it, physically, mentally, socially and ideologically, anywhere, at any time, and when he knows his human life on this planet is merely a process of the eternal cycle of change from infinity to the infinitesimal world, from the infinitesimal to infinity.

The way of practicing the order of the universe in our daily life, macrobiotics, shall guide all of us towards health and happiness, freedom and justice in this everlasting country of life in the infinite universe, and shall enable all of us to entertain ourselves in our endless play with our dream as present inhabitants on this small planet of Earth.

Levels of Judgment and Consciousness

Levels of Judgment		Name of Infinity in Each Level	Products in Each Level
7th Supreme	Universal and eternal consciousness. All-embracing, unconditional acceptance. Endless gratefulness, complete freedom.	Freedom	Eternal happiness with the spirit of One Grain, Ten Thousand Grains. Life in *Satori* or Nirvana.
6th Ideological	Distinction of justice and injustice, righteousness and unrighteousness.	Justice	Religions, doctrines, and disciplines.
5th Social	Distinction of good and bad, suitable and unsuitable, proper and improper, adaptability and inadaptability.	Peace	Ethics, moral codes, economy and politics.
4th Intellectual	Distinction of reason and unreason, proven and unproven.	Truth	Theory, concepts, organization, system.
3rd Sentimental	Distinction of love and hate, like and dislike, grace and awkwardness, joy and sadness.	Love	Arts, novels, poems, music.
2nd Sensory	Distinction of comfort and discomfort, full and hungry, beauty and ugliness.	Comfort and Pleasure	Tools, crafts, machines.
1st Mechanical	Spontaneous, automatic response.	Adaptability	Change is subject to the environmental stimulus.

Speaking in terms of time, any result of a mechanical response changes instantaneously. Spontaneous motion is a matter of seconds. The second, sensory result continues longer, but its remaining duration is a matter of minutes. The third sentimental feelings continue further, over a period of some days. The fourth intellectual theories can keep their influence over a duration of years. The fifth social ideas can last over a century. The sixth ideological products such as religions and doctrines, can last beyond a millenium. Spacewise, the lower judgment influences a fewer number of people, while the higher judgment gives wider influence upon a larger number of people and wider space. Yet, all results and influences produced by judgment from the first level to the sixth level are relative, ephemeral, and all disappear eventually, producing the opposite results. On the contrary, Supreme Judgment or Consciousness acts beyond the limits of time and space, and its influence is everlasting.

chapter 2

The Constitution of Man and His Food

Heaven has glorified Man; Earth has
inspired Woman. Both arose from the
ocean of antiquity. The destiny of
the human race goes together with
Heavenly motion and Earthly order.

December, 1976

1. The Emergence of Man

As most and possibly every phenomenon in this endless ocean of the infinite
universe tends to form a spirallic motion, including our galaxy, the Milky Way, all
appearances arising within our galaxy are therefore destined to move spirallically,
appearing and disappearing. The solar system, one of hundreds of millions of
similar systems belonging to this galaxy, may also form a spirallic motion in its
whole. The field of planets, including the orbits of Mercury, Venus, Earth, Mars,
Jupiter, Saturn, Neptune, Uranus and Pluto, is the nuclear region of the entire dimension of this system. Beyond this planetary region, more than 100,000,000 comets
are constantly running in an extended field approximately 3,850 times larger than
the field of planets—a dimension of about four light years. These orbits of millions
of comets may well be gradually turning towards the center of the system, destined
to enter into the planetary field through the change of their forms into planets.

Fig. 11   Spirallic Structure of the Milky Way and Solar System

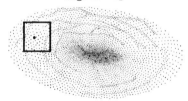

Oblique view of the Milky Way Galaxy.
Dot shows approximate position
of the solar system.

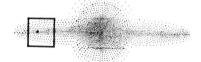

Side view of the Milky Way Galaxy.
Dot shows approximate position
of the solar system.

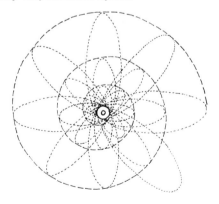

Schematic structure of the solar system.
Central circle shows the position of the
sun; next circle shows the planetary field;
spirallic petal design indicates various
orbits of comets.

Centripetal energy coming towards the sun turns its course towards the periphery and to the darkness far beyond the system in the form of solar winds and radiations. The sun may be a terminus of centripetality (yang) and the beginning of centrifugality (yin), rather than a shining body which is independent from the planets and comets. If it is so, the sun was born as a center of energy change, where the direction turns from incoming energy by combustion into outgoing heat, light, etc.

Within this organic solar system, nearly 4 billion years ago, our earth was a huge gaseous cloud. Within the cloud which was highly charged with intensive thunderstorms of electromagnetic activity, various light elements were produced: Hydrogen, Helium, Lithium, Beryllium, Boron, Carbon, Nitrogen and Oxygen. Fusions among them made further various heavier elements, and their combinations made various chemical compounds and molecules.

Elements, compounds and molecules heavier than others gradually gathered towards the center, eventually forming the solid part of the earth, while others of lighter weight gradually formed the periphery of the earth, eventually becoming the atmosphere. In between that solidifying matter and that expanding atmosphere, the water compound started to appear, and it covered the entire surface of the solid earth.

Within the storming gaseous cloud, primitive organic molecules—carbohydrates, proteins, virus, and bacteria—already began to appear, and continued to evolve mainly in the gradually forming water towards more highly evolved organisms. In general, out of the primary common molecule, two antagonistic-complementary streams of life began to evolve, namely the vegetable kindgom accelerated more by the centrifugal expanding force (yin), and the animal kingdom, stimulated more by the centripetal contracting force (yang). They continued to change, transform and differentiate into various species of life, mainly in water and later in air, over a period of more than 3.2 billion years of organic life, according to the change of environment.

In the water, during the Precambrian era, various water mosses in the kingdom of vegetables and various water invertebrates in the animal kingdom started to appear. Both the water vegetables and animals depended upon each other: the former as the food of the latter, the latter as nourishment to the former. This period may have continued nearly two billion years with gradual transformation of the organisms and their environment towards the next stage of development.

During this long period, the surrounding water gradually gathered a concentration of minerals, becoming salt water. Along with this yang process from water to salt water, the water plants were also changing more towards mineral-containing seaweeds, and the invertebrates transformed also, taking in minerals within their bodies, developing towards a variety of sea vertebrates, which are the ancestors of most of our present water animals. In this biological stage, evolution continued for approximately 0.8 billion years, as a latter course of the long development of water organisms, which is covering approximately 2.8 billion years as a whole. As a next great change, the land arose above the water, with repeated shattering of the earth. For the duration of millions of years in the progressive creation of land, water plants and animals were transported to the land, exposed to the air.

Some sea plants adapted to the land atmosphere, becoming land moss and primitive grasses. Some sea animals evolved towards amphibians which are able to live in both water and air. From them, evolution has taken place on the land, beginning approximately 400 million years ago.

As a next development in the progressive evolution of land species, a variety of ancient plants in the vegetable kingdom and a variety of primitive reptiles and birds in the animal kingdom began to appear about 200 million years ago. With the increasing temperature and humidity on the surface of the earth following that period and with the more intensified solar radiation, they grew eventually into the ancient giants—fern trees, horsetails, conifers, dinosaurs, flying reptiles, and others. Dominion of ancient plants as well as ancient birds and reptiles reached its zenith about 100 million years ago.

From that time the atmospheric temperature of the earth turned gradually colder. The age of modern plants, the ancestors of most present vegetables, and the age of mammals, depending upon these plants, began about 64 million years ago with the rapid extinction of the preceding giants. This biological modern age continued about 50 million years, during which most of the present species both in the vegetable kingdom and in the animal kingdom appeared. Their most prosperous time was about 40 million years ago.

As the earth continuously became colder, seed-bearing plants started to appear. The fruits and leaves which were once huge and juicy in the era of ancient plants, contracted in the colder climate, becoming smaller, harder and drier. Through this change of the vegetable kindgom, the species of apes expanded its varieties, eating these fruits, playing from tree to tree. In the field various herbaceous plants continuously produced smaller grains with harder shells as the climate became successively colder. The abundance of herbaceous grains was the beginning of the emer-

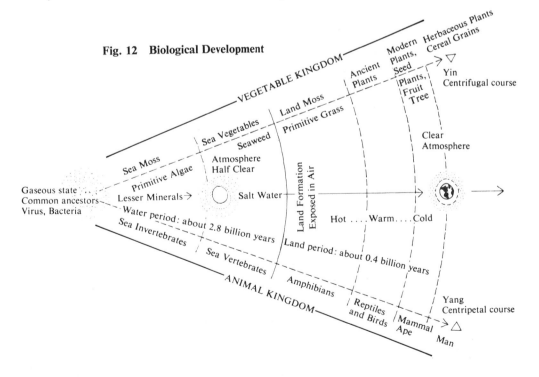

Fig. 12 Biological Development

gence of man through the eating of these grains, together with other preceding forms of life available in the surroundings. The time of the emergence of man may well be about 20 million years ago.

Since the time of the first emergence of man, the atmosphere of the earth has tended as a whole to become colder, with minor fluctuations alternating between warmer and cooler. In the most recent period of geological change, during a period of about one million years, the cycle of ice ages has begun in a more apparent pattern, with four great glacial and inter-glacial periods up to the present time. With these repeated periods of coldness, together with the eating of herbaceous grains and other plants, man could have developed an intelligence superior to any preceding animal species upon the earth.

Fig. 13   Four Ice Ages During Recent One Million Years

▽Glacial Period : Colder

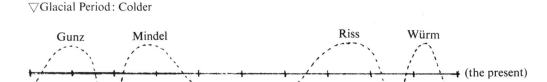

Gunz   Mindel   Riss   Würm

(the present)

△Interglacial Period : Warmer

The approximate alternation of glacial and interglacial periods during the past 1,000,000 years. First glacial—Gunz, 2nd glacial—Mindel, 3rd glacial—Riss, and 4th glacial—Würm.
The most recent 12,000 to 20,000 years is our present time.

As the cold climate covered a larger territory of the earth during the ice age, man began to use fire, using his intelligence to make him adaptable to the surroundings: first, applying to what he ate; second, applying to the production of tools and dwellings as well as clothing. The use of fire produced the birth of culture which led to the appearance of modern man, namely homo sapiens, and oriented his life towards the development of the prosperity of modern civilizations and cultures.

2. The Celestial Influence to Man

While biological life has progressed in its evolution for a period of more than 3.2 billion years, our solar system has been constantly running, with neighboring groups of similar systems orbiting around the center of our galaxy, the Milky Way. It is running at present with the speed of about 300 kilometers (186 miles) per second, making an entire orbit in about 200 million years. Though it may change gradually its duration of orbiting, we may assume that biological life has experienced more than 16 orbitings during its entire period of organic evolution.

In each orbiting, the distance from the center of our galaxy to our solar system may change from shorter to longer and longer to shorter. When it becomes shorter, the dimension of our solar system tends to slightly contract, resulting in the slight shortening of the distance between the sun and the earth. When it becomes longer, the solar system tends to become slightly expanded, resulting in the lengthening of the distance between the sun and the earth. During the shorter period, the earth receives more intensified solar radiation, becoming hotter and more wet in atmosphere, while during the longer period, it becomes colder and drier. This changing climate of the earth may well have produced the change of atmosphere which resulted in the gradual change of biological species.

About 100 million years ago on the muddy surface of the earth, ancient plants and animals flourished in their giant size. From that time, plants and animals have continuously become smaller and harder, up to the present time. Herbaceous plants and the human species are the appearance resulting from the cold climates in this orbiting cycle of galactic scale. Man is experiencing a colder climate than the time of the appearance of his preceding species such as the apes, mammals, reptiles and birds; and man will continuously experience increasing coldness for the future millions of years, with shorter cycles alternating between cold and warm climates. The reptiles and birds could be defined as the galactic spring-summer species; the mammals as autumn species; apes as late autumn and early winter; and man as the galactic winter species. How to eat his food and how to use fire in the preparation of food, are the matters of essence for the continual survival and development of the human species for millions of years in the future.

Furthermore, during more than 3.2 billion years of biological development, the atmosphere surrounding the earth has gradually changed from a heavy, dense gaseous state towards a light, clear state as it progressed. Celestial radiations from the sun, the moon, the planets, stars and galaxies, have showered upon the earth with more intensified varied radiations passing through the clearer atmosphere.

When the sun was the only shining celestial body sending its dim influence into the very ancient gaseous cloud of the earth, biological life was only single-celled beings. As the radiation from the moon and planets started to penetrate through the atmosphere of the earth, biological life began to differentiate into more cell divisions. As hundreds of thousands of stars began to send their various radiations,

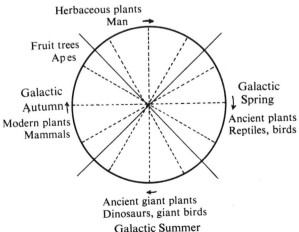

Fig. 14 Milky Way and Galactic Orbiting Cycle

The arrows show the direction of the solar system orbiting within the Milky Way Galaxy, taking approximately 200 million years—one Galactic Year—for one orbit. Each season is about 50 million years. Each dotted section, or galactic month, is approximately 16.6 million years. In the galactic summer, biological life becomes more expanded and cooler (cold-blooded), while in the galactic winter, it becomes contracted and warm-blooded. Man is a product of galactic winter.

more complex multi-cellular organisms began to evolve. As the millions of celestial bodies and their movements started to send influences even from the depths of the darkness of space, highly evolved plants and animals have come out.

The human constitution is reflecting its environment. Man's systems, organs and functions are reflecting and corresponding to the movement of groups of constellations and galaxies, as well as the influence of planetary movements. Without them, human life would not exist; and without their influence, the human body would not have its present form.

Fig. 15   The Celestial Constitution of Meridians

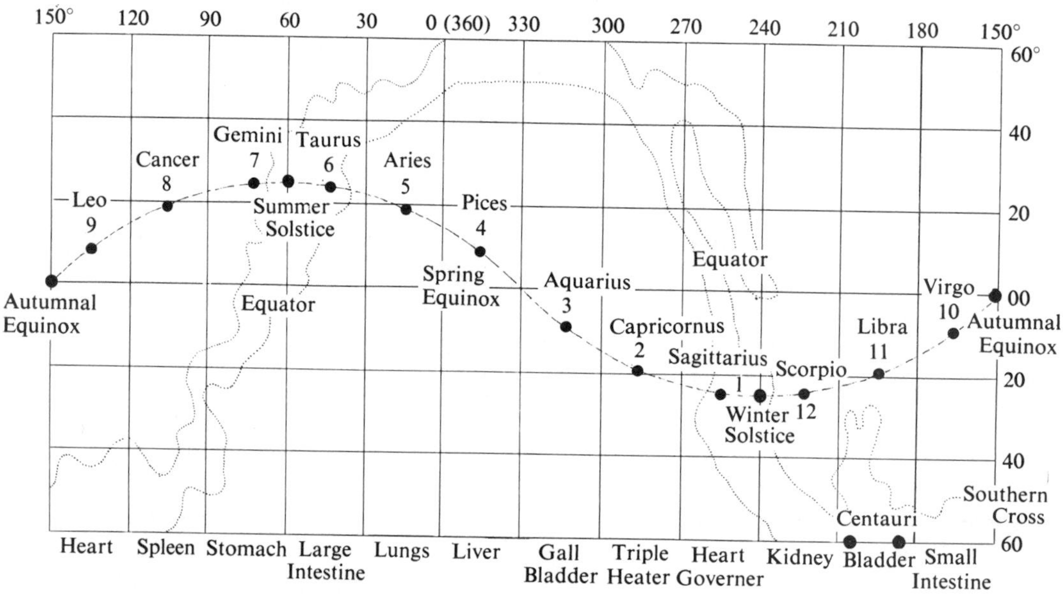

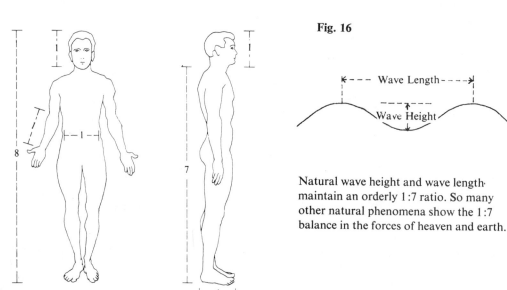

The force of celestial influence showering upon the earth day and night is seven times more than the expanding force accelerated by the rotation of the earth at present. Escaping velocity from the earth is seven while in other planets it varies. The natural formation of waves on the ocean shows a 7:1 ratio between the waves'

Fig. 16

Natural wave height and wave length maintain an orderly 1:7 ratio. So many other natural phenomena show the 1:7 balance in the forces of heaven and earth.

lengths and their heights. Recently-developed biological species, especially man, have a relation of head to body of 1:7. This ratio appears in the human structure in many aspects, as the average ideal proportion.

The ratio of 1:7 between the force of celestial influence, centripetal force, towards the center of the earth, and the expanding force generated by the motion of the earth, and in our human structure, suggest that our intake of physical environment in the form of food, drink, and breathing should be composed with this 1:7 ratio. Practically speaking, our consumption of the physical environment should be mineral to protein, 1:7; protein to carbohydrate, 1:7; carbohydrate to water, 1:7; water to air, 1:7 in their comparative weight. This, of course, varies according to the environment and individual condition, between 1:5 and 1:10.

Fig. 17   Solar Wind and Human Structure

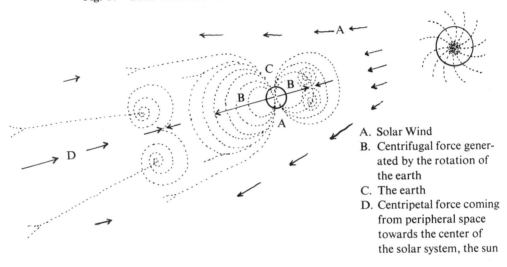

A. Solar Wind
B. Centrifugal force generated by the rotation of the earth
C. The earth
D. Centripetal force coming from peripheral space towards the center of the solar system, the sun

As the earth rotates, electromagnetic orbits are generated and formed around the earth. Towards these orbits, solar wind (A) from the sun and the centripetal force from the peripheral space (D) of the solar system, are coming, which collide with the centrifugal force generated by the earth's rotation (B), and form the human likeness of electromagnetic or plasmic energy.

By the practice of consuming food and other factors in this ratio, man is able to maintain maximum balance with his environment and can enjoy maximum flexibility in his activities. This is one of the important keys for everyone to achieve health and longevity.[1] Among many kinds of food available for man, unrefined whole cereal contains generally this ratio of minerals to protein, protein to carbohydrates.

---

[1] *Diet of the Hunza and Vilcabamba*
     In a survey of 55 adult males in Hunza, Pakistani nutritionist Dr. S. Maqsood Ali found an average caloric intake of 1,923 with 50 grams of protein, 36 grams of fat, and 354 grams of carbohydrate. Furthermore meat and dairy products constitute only 1–1/2 % of the total. The absence of pastureland makes animal husbandry nearly impossible, and the few livestock are usually killed for food during the festival season in winter. Fats of animal origin are scarce; instead, oil obtained from apricot seeds is generally used for all culinary purposes.
     "Dr. Guillermo Vela of Quito found a strikingly low caloric consumption also among the elderly▶

The ancient people called this celestial force coming to the earth and expanding force generated from the earth, the force of heaven and the force of earth, respectively. Everything and every phenomenon upon the surface of the earth is composed with those two forces, though some manifest more the force of heaven, appearing more contracted in shape, and others manifest more earth's force, appearing more expanded in size.

In the case of the human species, heaven's force enters more from the region of the top of the head, especially at the center of the hair spiral, moving downwards in the usual standing position. The force of the earth enters into the human body through the genital region going upward. Both forces are running as one channel, passing vertically through the most inner depths of the body. Both forces charge the five major areas in between on the way, producing seven major charging places in the body. Ancient Indians called them *chakras*.

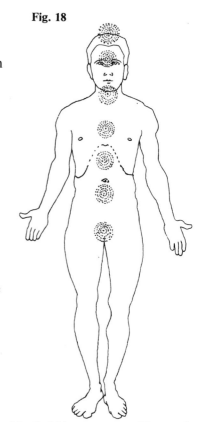

Fig. 18

Besides the hair spirallic region on the top of the head, and the genital region, being respectively the entrance and exit of heaven and earth forces, the five other chakras are: (1) the innermost region of the brain, namely the area of the midbrain, from which the charges are distributed to millions of brain cells. When the brain is charged, these brain cells are capable of receiving waves, interpreting them into images, and transmitting them as necessary responses—as the radio, television, computer, and other electromagnetic equipment are capable of doing similar work. (2) The region of the throat charging and activating the secretion of saliva, vibration of the uvula, and root of the tongue as well as the operation of the thyroid and parathyroid glands together with the rhythmical wave between inhaling and exhaling. (3) The third region charged by the heaven and earth forces is at the area of the heart, causing the formation of cardiac muscles and rhythmical motion of the heart between expansion and contraction, which operates throughout the circulatory system. (4) The fourth region is the stomach area from which charges are distributed to such organs in the middle trunk as the liver, spleen, pancreas and both kidneys, controlling and

▶of Vilcabamba. The average daily diet provided 1,200 calories. The daily protein intake was 35 to 38 grams, and of fat only 12 to 19 grams; 200 to 260 grams of carbohydrate completed the diet. Protein and fat again were largely of vegetable origin with only some 12 grams of protein daily from animal sources. Needless to say, one sees no obesity among the elderly in either Vilcabamba or Hunza; neither were there signs of undernutrition." (*National Geographic*, Vol. 143, No. 1, Jan. 1973, "Every Day Is A Gift When You Are Over 100" by Alexander Leaf, M. D.)

directing the operation of their rhythmical functions. (5) The fifth region is the center of the intestinal area, the so-called TAN-DEN (丹田) or HARA (肚), the inner depths below the navel, the central area to maintain body equilibrium—charge from this area is distributed to all parts of the small and large intestines as well as to the bladder and genital areas, making active and rhythmical operation of the digestion, decomposition, and absorption of food, water and energy.

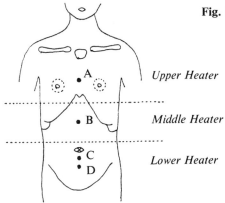

Fig. 19   The Triple Heater

Upper Heater

Middle Heater

Lower Heater

A. DAN-CHU (膻中)—CV17
B. CHU-KANG (中脘)—CV12
C. IN-KO (陰交)—CV7
D. KI-KAI (気海)—CV6

In oriental medicine, three regions, represented by the heart, stomach, and intestine, are called SAN-SHO (三焦)—Triple Heater—three regions of generating heat. Each of these regions has respectively central points as listed at left; these are the central places of the three chakras and are used for diagnosis and treatment in acupuncture, moxibustion, shiatsu, massage, and palm healing.

The functions of these chakras are respectively governing various physiological and mental activities in each region. However, internally these chakras are vitalized by the stream of blood which is also charged electromagnetically. Therefore, depending upon the volume and quality of the consumption of food and drink as well as the speed and frequency of breathing activity, the function of the chakras changes. Hence, to change consciousness or to develop physical coordination, to achieve physical, mental and spiritual development, the principle of how to consume our environment in the form of food, drink, breath and consciousness is of the utmost importance. All spiritual, religious, and social disciplines as well as physical exercises began from this understanding.[2]

---

[2] In the practice of meditation there are many techniques to emphasize and activate certain chakras. Also, basic meditation is aiming to smooth heaven's and earth's forces passing through an inharmonious state. Zen meditation mainly emphasizes HARA while some other meditations emphasize more the midbrain.

All monasteries, temples and shrines as well as many physical, mental, and spiritual training places have practiced dietary disciplines such as SHOJIN RYORI (精進料理), "cuisine for spiritual advancement," in the case of Buddhism, and unleavened bread with vegetables in the Christian monasteries, and the practice of Kasruth among Jewish tradition. Founders and originators of various martial arts and great philosophers and thinkers in old times all practiced dietary disciplines—which are all along the macrobiotic way.

3. Man Can Eat Everything

Man, as the last and most recent development of the animal kingdom upon the earth, has taken in within himself all preceding qualities of various animal species. Accordingly, man is capable of eating and taking in within himself all levels of the animal world in the form of food. Biologically speaking, eating a preceding animal species is the process of evolution shortened in its period, from the less developed species to more highly developed ones. In this sense, when man eats animal food, these animal species become a part of man.[3] Eating more primitive lives and being eaten by more developed beings are processes of evolution repeating and accomplishing with very rapid speed the entire evolution of over three billion years from protozoa to highly developed forms, from a single-cell organism to a complex being. For example, through being eaten and digested, protozoa transform into a part of the fish. Through the same process, fish become a part of the flying seagulls. Flying birds, being eaten by beasts, become the beasts running in the fields; and when beasts are eaten by man, they become man. On the contrary, if the lower species devour highly evolved species, this process is degeneration of life. When we are eaten by other mammals or mosquitoes as well as bacteria and virus, our human status is not proper as mankind, and we progress towards rapid degeneration.

Many modern men are eating a variety of mammal species: cows in the form of beef; pigs in the form of ham and bacon; goats in the form of lamb; and their products in the form of milk, cheese and other dairy food. Man also eats from the ancient animal species, many birds and reptiles such as chicken, turkey, duck, and pheasant, with their eggs, as well as snakes and lizards. Among amphibious species, man eats frogs and their legs, turtles, snails and many others. Among fish swimming in the ocean and river, a plentiful variety of fish: salmon, eel, tuna, mackerel, snapper, trout, haddock, cod, sole, etc.; out of invertebrates living in the water, various shellfish, squid, octopus and many others. Man further eats the most primordial life —bacteria, enzymes and various forms of virus in and within all sorts of fermented and processed food, as well as in the water and in the air.

The fact that man is capable of eating and taking in most of those preceding animal species, either in part or in their entirety, also suggests that he can eat most vegetable species which are nothing but the original form of animal species, considering that the animal species ate them—even in the carnivorous animal who eats only other animals, the animals they eat are eating vegetables, and therefore the meat-eating animals are in fact eating reprocessed vegetables.[4]

---

[3] "Jesus said: Blessed is the lion which the man eats and the lion will become man; and cursed is the man whom the lion eats and the man will become lion." (From the *Gospel According to Thomas*, Log. 7, pub. 1959 by Harper and Row, Trans. by Guillaumont, Puech, Quispel, Till and Yassah 'Abd Al Masih.—p. 5.)

[4] Among modern vegetarianism, one of the reasons supporting vegetarianism is that killing is not ethical. However, this reason is merely based upon sentimentality for the reason that (1) all vegetable plants also have lives, and (2) we observe as the natural course that the highly developed species eat less developed species. Such sentimental reasoning to support vegetarianism as a whole comes from a lack of understanding of the order of the universe.

Man, universally, eats all kinds of grain products among the cereal and legume plants, such as rice, wheat, millet, oats, barley, rye, corn, buckwheat, as well as soybeans, lima beans, kidney beans, chickpeas, lentils, split peas and many others. Among biologically recent plants, he eats various seeds, fruits and nuts. Man eats also many modern vegetables, including watercress, kale, carrots, turnips, potatoes, squash, pumpkin, radish, cabbage, Chinese cabbage, onions, scallions and others. He also eats ancient-origin plants such as ferns, asparagus, and many fungi such as mushrooms. Man further eats sea plants: *kombu, wakame, hijiki,* dulse, Irish moss and *nori.* He further eats the most primitive plant life—molds, yeast and the like.

Man is really a universal eater. Man is the most capable among all animal species of eating so many varieties of food. Modern man has added in his food even artificially processed and synthesized food, chemicalized, industrialized and mass-produced food. Moreover, man changes the quality of food in various degrees by applying methods of processing, choosing, combining, preserving, and cooking with the additional treatment of drying and watering, pickling, pressuring, heating and freezing, storing and fermenting.

If we eat more variety, the result is our greater biological development; if we eat less variety, that creates less biological development. Also, a society whose people are applying more developed cooking becomes more culturally developed, while a society whose people apply more primitive cooking becomes less developed.

Through the ages as man has been learning more well-developed ways of choosing, preparing and cooking foods, he has been able to create cultures which are more developed. When we see cooking methods in a household, we can know its family's state of mind; and when we see the general way of cooking in one country or race, we can know their mental and spiritual stage.

While man can eat almost all biological life—animal and vegetable species—man also eats and drinks minerals and water. Almost all elements exist in different degrees within his body, and 80% of the human body consists of water. He takes these substances in the form of vegetable and animal food as well as in the form of salts, refined and unrefined, and he takes many varieties of liquid in the form of juicy fruits, vegetables, cooked grains and flours, and in the form of soup and beverage. In other words, man eats every day a part of his natural environment upon the earth which is manifesting in the form of mineral, liquid, and biological life.

Responding to those parts of his physical environment which he eats, he further takes in air, especially oxygen (O_2), eliminating a part of the used food in the form of carbon dioxide (CO_2). The intake of air is proportional to the quality and volume of what he eats out of the mineral, liquid and biological worlds. The more he eats, the more he breathes; the less he eats, the less he breathes. The more animal food he eats, the more inhaling increases; the more vegetable quality food he eats, the more harmonious breathing becomes.[5]

---

[5] "*Respiratory Quotient* (*RQ*): This is the ratio of the volume of CO_2 produced and oxygen (O_2) consumed, expressed as follows:

$$\frac{\text{Volume of } CO_2 \text{ expired}}{\text{Volume of } O_2 \text{ inspired}} = \text{Respiratory Quotient}$$

▶

When he eats a certain variety of food, a certain quality of blood starts to stream. When he eats certain other varieties, a certain other quality of blood streams. However small the difference may be, a pinch of sea salt, a few drops of soy sauce, a slice of cheese, a few sections of orange, a half teaspoonful of sugar, a cup of tea, delicately change the quality and volume of blood. When the quality and volume of blood change, the quality of cells and body as a whole including brain and nervous system change automatically. These changes transform physical and psychological functions, influencing all behavior and expressions. Physical movement and habits, as well as sensory perception, emotional response, intellecutal conception, social consciousness and philosophical view of life are changing day to day because of the change in what we consume.

Like a television having inferior parts and unable to receive and transmit into images and sound a series of vibrations coming from a distant station, if our blood is inferior, we are unable to perceive and respond to waves and vibrations coming from short and long distances. If our consciousness is sometimes clouded, it may be due to the change of environmental vibrations; but it is more largely due to what we are taking into our body by ourselves. We understand when we see that some person may react nervously but another person maintains normal response under the same circumstances, which explains that psychological variations are largely owing to what we consume daily.

We are what we eat, and we are totally responsible ourselves for our physical and mental condition. Whether we are active, healthy and happy or inactive, sick or

---

▶ In the oxidation of a carbohydrate, the following reaction takes place:
$$C_6H_{12}O_6 + 6O_2 \rightarrow 6CO_2 + 6H_2O \quad \text{plus energy}$$
Then,

$$\frac{6 \text{ volumes of } CO_2}{6 \text{ volumes of } O_2} = 1.0 \quad \text{(RQ of a carbohydrate)}$$

Similarly, the RQ for a fat is 0.71; for a protein, it is 0.80. For a person on an average mixed diet, it is 0.85. For a person who has fasted for 12 hours, the RQ is 0.82. "(From *Anatomy and Physiology*, Vol. I by Steen and Montagu, Harper & Row, 1959, p. 195.) RQ indicates that if we eat animal food in large volume, which consists of much protein and fat, more rapid and rough breathing is required, which influences our mind, more disturbing from normal quietness. Accordingly, those who practice meditation and other spiritual exercises should avoid a consumption of large amounts of animal food.

"He who knows this (as described above), after dying to (i.e., withdrawing from) this world, attains the self which consists of food, attains the self which consists of the vital breath, attains the self which consists of the mind, attains the self which consists of the intellect, attains the self which consists of bliss. Then he goes up and down these worlds, eating the food he desires, assuming the forms he likes. He sits, singing the chant of the non-duality of Brahman: 'Ah! Ah! Ah!'

'I am food, I am food, I am food! I am the eater of food, I am the eater of food, I am the eater of food! I am the uniter, I am the uniter, I am the uniter!

'I am the first-born of the true, prior to the gods, and the navel of Immortality. He who gives me away, he alone preserves me. He who eats food— I, as food, eat him.

'I (as the Supreme Lord) overpower the whole world. I am radiant as the sun.'

Whosoever knows this (attains Liberation). Such, indeed, is the Upanishad." (III.x. 6)

(From the *Taittiriya Upanishad*)

unhappy, on this earth, depends entirely upon ourselves and no one else. We are always the master of ourselves, and no one else can really control our personal destiny. Miserable sickness and death, dark frustration and suffering, severe accidents and failures, are all caused in ourselves, coming from what we choose as our food, according to whether such food is suitable in our environment. The secret for health and wisdom, freedom and happiness—all physical, mental and spiritual as well as all social well-being—is in front of us, day-to-day, lying in every dish we consume. How to choose, how to prepare, how to eat are the most central answers to the questions of the destiny of man—personal and collective, for the individual and for entire mankind. Man can eat everything, and yet he must maintain a certain order in what he consumes. That is a turning point to direct him towards development or decline.

4. Food of Embryo and Infant

Both man and woman receive constantly the celestial influence, heaven's force, which is moving downwards towards the earth, and centrifugal force, the earth's force, generated by the movement of the rotation of the earth. These forces are running through both man's and woman's body independently when they are separated, but when man and woman meet together, the flow of these forces becomes more intensified by connecting their magnetic poles of these forces, which are the sexual organs. At that time, the male reproductive cell, the sperm (yin), fuses with the female reproductive cell, the ovum (yang), and fertilization and implantation occurs at the place of one of the chakras in the female body, the HARA or TAN-DEN, the inner depths of the uterus. This occurrence is repeating the primordial period of creation of the organism in the very ancient gaseous state of the earth, far beyond three billion years ago.

From that time, the fertilized egg develops towards the embryonic state progressively in the surrounding of fluid within the amnion. The first period of three months forms the structural systems, namely the inner digestive and respiratory systems, the outer nervous systems and central circulatory and excretory systems (refer to earlier diagram, Chapter One). Organs and glands are also developed along these systems during this period. The following period of pregnancy sees the development in the embryo of various auxiliary parts of the body together with growth as a whole, until the end of the embryonic period.

This entire embryonic period, approximately 280 days, is a repetition of the evolutional process of biological life in the ocean of the earth, until the time of the rise of land upon the surface of the water. This embryonic period, accordingly, repeats at least 2.8 billion or nearly 3 billion biological years for the period of 280 days. The average speed of growth is 10 million biological years per each 24 hours, and the similar takes place in the increase of body weight, which reaches 6 to 8 pounds at the time of delivery, from very minor weight in the beginning of pregnancy, an increase of almost 3 billion times. Therefore, it is understandable that the quality and volume of food intake at that period through the mother's blood and placenta is giving a determining influence to the structure and quality of the human constitution. Even though the DNA molecule in the chromosomes together with the RNA molecules are carrying numerous hereditary factors, the influence of food intake is essential to secure smooth development. The constitution developed in the embryonic age is the foundation for the entire human life after the birth to this world, until the time of death.

During her conception and gestation period, if the mother lives with peaceful thoughts, active life, and with the proper environment and food, the coming birth is smooth and rapid, and she can enjoy natural birth without the need of any medical and artificial assistance. A baby who is born smoothly through natural birth has the native potentiality to grow healthy and active in his physical and mental life. However, if the mother nourishes the baby within her uterus with the improper quality and volume of food, the newborn life would suffer in the process of growing in the uterus, and often there would be structural deformation or mental retardation resulting as well. Even without noticeable differences in form and function, the baby would have a potential weakness for physical, mental and social abilities, which would continue throughout his life. Many so-called hereditary diseases or causes of physical and mental sicknesses which may be suffered during the growing period towards adulthood, are planted in the improper thought and food consumption as well as unnatural style of living of the mother and of the parents as a unit.

From ancient times, the importance of the pregnancy period as a foundation of the entire life has been well known among traditional people. In the Orient they practiced Tai-Kyo (胎教), embryonic education, which was aiming to produce a better quality of baby, physically healthy and mentally happy, through the behavior

Fig. 20 Deformations

These three deformations are caused by the inability to contract, due to insufficient minerals or excessive intake of fluid during the period of pregnancy, through the mother's dietary practice. These deformations, and many others as well, are increasing as modern dietary habits are becoming more disorderly.

Harelip   Hydrocephalus   Webbed Fingers

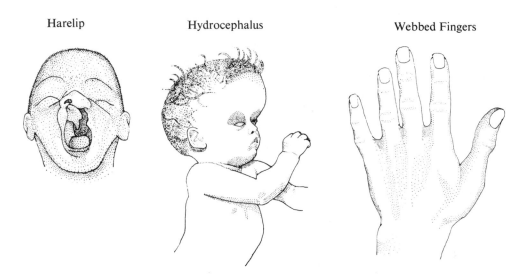

of the parents and especially the mother. For all parents, it is highly recommended to practice the following:

1. To maintain peaceful and happy relations among parents and family members, avoiding quarrels and conflicts.
2. To wear simple, neat clothing, preferably of vegetable quality such as cotton, at least for underwear, and to keep them clean and sanitary.
3. To keep the household in order, and to keep every part of the house clean and orderly.
4. To avoid activities or experiences which may stimulate unnecessary excitement —disturbances such as seeing violent scenes and monstrous pictures or hearing loud disturbing music and sounds.
5. To keep energetic activity in daily life, either keeping the household or through working, until the very end of the pregnancy period.

Furthermore, parents, especially the mother, should follow the proper dietary practices. Cereal grains, beans, and land and sea vegetables are always for daily consumption, but the mother may need additional consumption of fruits, seeds, nuts and a small amount of animal food, according to necessity.[6]

The time of delivery is a repeating of the natural event of the shattering of the earth experienced approximately 400 million years ago. The land rose together with vast floods by recurring great earthquakes, as the ancient sea animals were transferred upon the land. Similarly, the delivery brings a baby from the water surroundings to the air environment, together with a flow of water. The baby rapidly adapts to the new environment, contracting his physical body by means of the contraction of the uterus as he passes through the narrow birth channel. He cries out excessive gas, and a few days of fasting following the birth complete his contraction process. After that process of contraction, he begins the experience of biological evolution as land animal, towards man. The baby passes similar stages of amphibian, reptile, mammal and ape, gradually standing from preceding curved postures towards the perfect postural erection as a human infant. When he stands and becomes equipped with infant teeth, he has achieved the entire process of biological evolution, approximately 3.2 billion years, covering water and land life as well.

During this period of pregnancy and after the moment of birth, up to the development of erect posture as a human infant, the baby is continuously eating food of animal quality. This period is divided into two: before and after delivery. Before delivery, the food the baby takes through the placenta and umbilical cord is permeated with the mother's blood, the most condensed form of animal substance, in order to accomplish the entire biological evolution in the ocean-like environment for the duration of only nine months. After the delivery, the food changes into a sweeter and more diluted animal liquid, the mother's milk, in order to accomplish biolog-

---

[6] There are many traditional sayings in connection with TAI-KYO (embryonic education). For example: (1) "Do not feed eggplant to a new bride." (2) "A married woman should avoid eating meat and eggs." (3) "A household which has a fig tree in the back yard will perish by not having offspring." (4) "When you want to know a person, see his mother." These sayings are teaching us about the long experience of dietary importance.

ical evolution upon the land environment in generally about a one-year period.

As mentioned before, embryonic development goes on the average at a rate of 10 million biological years each day, covering approximately 2.8 billion biological years in ocean life followed by 400 million biological years on the land—this entire scope of development taking place in less than a one-year period after birth. The quality of the food which the baby takes during these two periods gives an absolutely essential influence to the formation of the constitution and destiny for the entire life thereafter. For example, in the event the mother takes a tranquilizer or unusual chemical during her pregnancy, it may well be changing for several days the quality of the fluid in the amnion, and the blood in the embryo that the baby absorbs. That means, the baby is living in polluted surroundings with heavily contaminated food. In the same manner, while the baby is taking mother's milk, if he is given improper quality of baby food artificially and chemically produced, or even if he is given cow's or goat's milk, the development of the baby towards proper human infancy is disturbed in considerable degree. This consideration would reveal a clear answer for many cases of deformation and other congenital defects, and weak constitution. The happiness of man and what he does and enjoys in his life are really largely depending upon the way of eating during these periods.[7]

5. Food for Human Beings

Upon the achievement of the biological growing process from a single-celled fertilized egg to the multicellular evolved human infant, man has actually completed his eating of animal food. The animal food was necessary to shorten the process of development from the undeveloped animal species into higher species. However,

---

[7] *Human Milk versus Cow's Milk*: Milk is an emulsion of fat particles suspended in a watery fluid containing proteins, sugar (especially lactose), and inorganic salts. A comparison of human milk and cow's milk is seen in the following table:

Substance	Human Milk	Cow's Milk
Water	88.3%	87.3
Inorganic salts	0.2	0.7
Protein	1.5	3.8
Fat	4.0	4.0
Sugars	6.0	4.5
Reaction	Alkaline	Acid

"Human milk is regarded as definitely superior to cow's milk or other foods in the following respects: (1) It is cleaner and freer from bacteria. (2) Its composition varies during the first few weeks of lactation, in accordance with the varying needs of the infant. (3) Its protein is principally soluble lactalbumin instead of the relatively insoluble caseinogen of cow's milk. The curd formed in the stomach from human milk is therefore less dense and is more readily digested. (4) The fat is in a more finely emulsified form, and there is a smaller proportion of fatty acids. (5) The percentage of lactose is higher. (6) Immune bodies from the mother's blood induce a greater degree of immunity in the infant. (7) Breast-fed babies, in contrast to bottle-fed babies, suffer less frequently from disturbances of the gastrointestinal tract (diarrhea, for example) and they recover more quickly from postnatal birth-weight loss." (From *Anatomy and Physiology*, Vol. 2, by Steen and Montagu, Barnes & Noble, 1959, p. 253.)

when we reach the stage of human beings, we should start to consume human food, which consists of various species of the vegetable kingdom, the origin of all animal species. Man, therefore, should eat cereal grains as his daily principal food and various land vegetables as his secondary food, sea vegetables with primordial seawater as his third food, and if he wants to include in his consumption some animal quality, species that are more primordial than the highly evolved ones can be the next category of his food. This means, fowl is more recommended than mammals such as beef and pork; fish and other seafood are more suitable than fowl such as chicken or turkey. This suggests that if daily foods include animal quality, water animals would be the most preferable and land animals would be the least preferable.

In the biological process of evolution, the period of water life, approximately 2.8 billion years, vs. the period of land life, approximately 0.4 billion years, is about 7 to 1 in ratio. Since we are the last land development, the composition of our food should be reversed—generally land quality seven parts, and water quality one part. This further suggests that if we include animal food, preferably a variety of fish and seafood, all vegetable quality food vs. animal quality food should be in a ratio of less than 7:1.

Fig. 21   Principle of Food According to Biological Evolution

Category A to B, condensed in the form of mother's blood and of mother's milk, is embryonic and infant food. Category C to D is the food for man after he becomes a human infant, for the development of his humanhood. Throughout those two periods we eat the entire biological scope.

The second supplemental food, seaweed and sea moss, with or without the third supplemental food—fish and seafood—can be in the form of soup, especially using bacteria and enzymes, the most primordial life, in the form of fermented seasoning.

Fruits and nuts can be served only as a supplement to the entire meal. Cereal grains are fruits of herbaceous plants, and therefore when man is eating cereal grains he does not need to eat additional fruits in the main part of his meal.

If we choose animal food, we should choose that animal food which is further from us in terms of species.

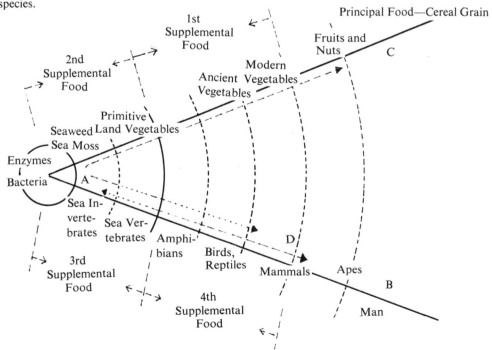

Our adult teeth as we easily may examine ourselves, consist as follows:

Fig. 22

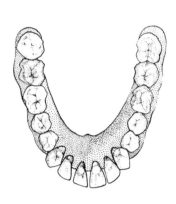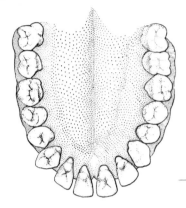

Incisors .... 8 teeth
Canines .... 4 teeth
Pre-molars and
    molars ....20 teeth
Total ......32 teeth

The majority of our teeth, pre-molars and molars, generally suggest their use for grain grinding—cereals, legumes, and other seed grains. The second largest number of teeth, incisors, suggest vegetable cutting and the least number of teeth, canines, are primarily for tearing animal food. This arrangement of use is of course very general, and yet we can see the principal food should be grains and the second, vegetables; the third, and last, animal quality food. According to our teeth arrangement, the general ratio of grain to vegetables to animal food would be 5:2:1, and all vegetable quality to animal quality, 7:1. Furthermore, some people do not have pointed canines while others have more pointed ones. This fact is indicating that the eating of animal food is rather optional than a requirement to maintain human life.

From the above view of biological development upon this earth, our daily meal is recommended to be composed as follows, according to the order of volume:

1.   50% or more whole cereal grains and their products—representing present

---

Ten Days of Eating Pulse
"But Daniel purposed in his heart that he would not be defiled with the king's table, nor with the wine which he drank: and he requested the master of the eunuchs that he might not be defiled. And God gave to Daniel grace and mercy in the sight of the prince of the eunuchs. And the prince of the eunuchs said to Daniel: I fear my lord the king, who hath appointed you meat and drink: who if he should see your faces leaner than those of the other youths your equals, you shall endanger my head to the king. And Daniel said to Malasar, whom the prince of the eunuchs had appointed over Daniel, Ananias, Mesael, and Azarius: Try, I beseech thee, thy servants for ten days, and let pulse be given us to eat, and water to drink. And look upon our faces, and the faces of the children that eat of the king's meat: and as thou shalt see, deal with thy servants. And when he had heard these words, he tried them for ten days. And after ten days their faces appeared fairer and fatter than all the children that ate of the king's meat. So Malasar took their portions, and the wine that they should drink: and he gave them pulse. And to these children God gave knowledge and understanding in every book, and wisdom: but to Daniel the understanding also of all visions and dreams."

(Pulse=grains.)

The Old Testament, The Book of Daniel, Ch. I, 8–17.

vegetable species.
2. 10%–15% beans, seeds and their products—representing recent biological species.
3. 25% land and sea vegetables as well as soup, ancient seawater—representing modern, ancient and primordial ages of the sea.
4. Less than 15% animal food—representing animal quality parallel to the above.
5. An occasional use of fruit and fruit products in small volume—representing recent biological species before grains.
6. The most primordial biological life, enzymes and bacteria, necessary for our consumption, may be also supplemented in the form of fermented food in small volumes—representing the most primordial age of biological life.

Therefore, in the actual preparation of the meal, food can be categorized into the principal food and supplemental food in normal climates where most of the world's population lives (excepting the very cold polar regions):

Principal Foods:

These are the essential foods and central portion for daily consumption, and are to be eaten at every meal as the main dish.

A. *Cereal grains and similar:* brown rice, whole wheat, barley, oats, rye, millet, corn, buckwheat. (Corn and buckwheat are not, strictly speaking, cereal species, but can be treated as such.)

B. *Legumes and seeds:*
Beans: *azuki* beans, chickpeas, lentils, kidney beans, pinto beans, navy beans, black beans, soy beans, split peas, and others.
Seeds: sesame seeds, sunflower seeds, pumpkin seeds, chia seeds, and many others.

Supplemental Foods:

All other food not belonging to the principal food category are considered as supplemental food, which altogether should make up less than 50% in volume of daily consumption.

A. *Land Vegetables*
1. *More modern species and temperate origin:*
Daikon (long white radish), radish, carrots, burdock, parsnip, salsify, and their leaves, cabbage, Chinese cabbage, lettuce, spinach, kale, watercress, parsley, Swiss chard, bok choy, collard greens, mustard greens, celery, cucumber, summer squash, autumn squash, pumpkin, onion, leek, scallion, green peas, stringbeans, mountain potato (*jinenjo*), dandelion, clover, grain and bean sprouts, and many others.
2. *More ancient and tropical species:*
Potato, sweet potato, yam, tapioca, tomato, eggplant, asparagus, green pepper, artichoke, bamboo shoot, okra, beets, lotus root, and many others.
3. *More primitive origin:*
Mushroom and many other vegetables belonging to the fungi species.

B. *Sea Vegetables*—Seaweeds and sea moss:
Wakame and its sprout, *kombu* and its sprout, *hijiki*, *nori*, dulse, Irish moss, agar-agar, *arame*, and many others.

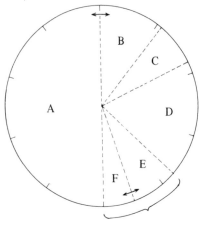

With Animal Food

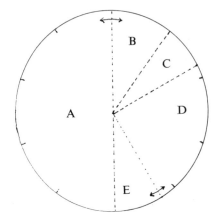

Vegetable Quality Only

Fig. 23   Dietary Proportions in View of Biological Development

A. Whole cereal grains
B   Legumes, seeds
C. Soup, representing ancient seawater, with sea salt, enzymes or bacteria, and sea vegetables.
D. Vegetables: ancient, modern, and sea vegetables
E. Animal food, preferably fish and seafood, or primitive land animal
F. Fruits and nuts

A. Whole cereal grains
B. Legumes, seeds
C. Soup, representing ancient seawater, with sea salt, enzyme or bacteria, and sea vegetables
D. Vegetables: ancient, more cooked, and modern, less cooked
E. Fruits and nuts, as well as raw modern vegetables and pickles

Arrows show interchange and flexibility among neighboring categories.

C. *Fruits and Nuts:*
1. *Temperate zone fruits:*   Apples, cherries, peaches, plums, apriocot, strawberries, blueberries, blackberries and other berries, canteloupe, honeydew melon, watermelon and other melons, grapes, mandarin oranges, and many others.
2. *Tropical fruits:*   Oranges, lemons, limes, pineapple, coconut, mango, papaya, banana, avocado, casaba melon, and many others.
3. *Temperate and tropical nuts:*   Almonds, walnuts, pecans, filberts, peanuts, cashews, Brazil nuts, pine nuts, and many others.

D. *Animal Food*
1. *Water species—fish and seafood:*
   Fish: Sole, halibut, hake, cod, salmon, trout, scrod, sea trout, red snapper, bluefish, whitefish, flounder, haddock, smelt, carp, swordfish, tuna, snapper, mackerel, sardine, anchovy, eel, and many others, as well as their eggs.
   Seafood: Oyster, clam, scallop, mussel, shrimp, lobster, crab, and many others.

Question: How about dairy food, honey, and nuts?
Answer: They are so wonderful and properly nutritious— milk for cows. honey for bees, nuts for squirrels. But when man eats them, he should be wise how much volume and in what way he takes them.

2. *Amphibious species:* Frog, snail, turtle and many others, as well as their eggs.
3. *Reptile and bird species:* Snake, lizard, chicken, turkey, pheasant, partridge, and others, as well as their eggs.
4. *Mammal species:* Rabbit, boar, horse, dog, cat, squirrel, pig, sheep and many others, as well as goats and cows, their milk and milk products.

E. *Enzymes and Bacteria*

Natural enzymes and bacteria can be produced during the process of digestion but in order to make digestive and absorbing functions smoothly activated, many fermented foods and beverages have been used. For example:

1. *Vegetable-base quality:* Miso, *tamari* soy sauce, *koji* (molded grain), *natto*, sauerkraut and other pickles, and many others.
2. *Animal-base quality:* Cheese, yoghurt, buttermilk, and others.
3. *Beverages:* Beer, whisky, wine, and many other fermented alcoholic beverages.

However, the actual way of preparation and eating of these foods should be followed according to the following principles considered from, again, a process of biological evolution:

1. *Principal food*, namely cereal grains, and their products—such as bread, chapati, noodles and pasta—from the beginning to the end of the meal. Beans and seeds, since they are near to the cereal species, could be used also as a part of the principal food, or with the dish of principal food. For example, beans could be cooked or served together with rice and other grains; and sesame seeds together with sea salt roasted and crushed, can be used as a condiment for the dish of grain.
2. *Soup*, consisting of sea vegetables with or without fish flavor, and sometimes including land vegetables, beans or grains, is to be served as the first portion of side dishes. Such soup, especially containing sea vegetables and fermented enzymes with slightly salty taste, is actually a condensed form of the ancient sea within which early life evolved before the formation of land
3. *Land vegetable dishes*, containing leafy, ground, and root vegetables, cooked in various forms, such as sauteeing, steaming, boiling, baking, and frying (when we use oil, it should be of vegetable quality)—to be served as the second part of side dishes. Vegetables of more ancient origin should be cooked more, and those of more recent origin may be cooked less and may be occasionally taken in uncooked form such as salad or pickles, according to environmental conditions and personal need.
4. *Seaweeds and water moss* cooked separately or together with some land vegetables or beans—can be served as the third part of side dishes. These seaweeds and water mosses can be served in soup as the first part of side dishes.
5. *Fish, seafood and other animal food*, if required—can be taken as part of the second part of side dishes, together with land and sea vegetables, because of their complementary and antagonistic relation in biological development. However, as mentioned before, more primordial animal life is preferred.
6. *Fruits and nuts*, chosen locally according to season, may be the last course of

side dishes or last supplement to the entire meal, which may be occasionally taken as dessert either in fresh, cooked or dried form in the case of fruits, and roasted with sea salt in the case of nuts.

7. *Beverage*—as a last part of the entire meal, may be taken together with dessert or alone when required. Such beverage usually should be made of modern herb plants but occasionally could be made of ancient plants and sea vegetables. However, such fermented beverages as alcoholic beverages may be taken in small volume before the meal if the first part of side dishes is not soup containing fermented enzymes, to smooth appetite and digestion.

Fig. 24   The Order of Eating

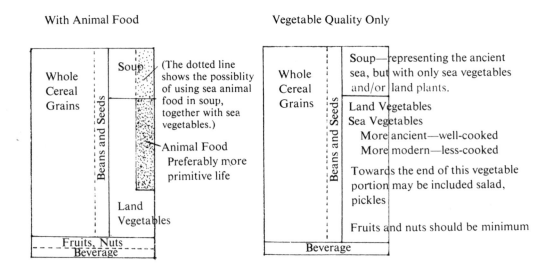

Shaded area indicates the proportion of animal food, which should be less than 15% of the entire meal.

The order of eating goes from top to bottom. We begin with soup, together with cereal grains. Animal food must be stopped part way through the meal, finishing with vegetable quality. Last—dessert, beverage. (Dotted lines within each section of the diagrams show that it is possible to interchange flexibly with the neighboring category.)

Geological Change and Biological Development

Era and Period		Geological Change	Botanical Change	Zoological Change
		Formation of the Earth No organic life		
I	Antiquitic Era (Duration: unknown)	Gaseous Heavy, thick environment	Transferring from inorganic molecule to organic molecule through thunder- storms and electromagnetic activity Carbohydrate and protein molecule	
. . . . about 2.2 billion years ago				
		Water appearance	Virus-bacteria	
II	Archeozoic Era (Duration: about 2.2 billion years)	Atmosphere still heavier and darker	Single-cell beings	
		Water progressively changes to higher mineral content	Flagellates	Water primordial animal life
———— about 1 billion years ago				
		Atmosphere— more clear	Water moss	Sea invertebrates
III	Proteozoic Era (Duration: about 500 million years)	Ocean water— more salty Salt water	Various algae Seaweed	Sea vertebrates
———— about 500 million years ago				

IV	Paleozoic Era Cambrian Period
	  Ordovician Period
	(Duration: about Silurian Period
	330 million yrs.) Devonian Period
	  Carboniferous Period
	  Perneian Period
		Land formation
		
		Continental division
		and shift progress
			Algae fossils
			
			Land moss
			Fungi and primor-
			dial land plants
				Amphibians
				Land worms
				Primitive insects

———— about 170 million years ago				
V	Mesozoic Era (Duration: about Triassic Period 110 million yrs.) Jurassic Period Cretaceous Period	Frequent volcanic activity Muddy surface	Ancient plants Ancient seed plants	Reptiles and birds
———— about 60 million years ago				
VI	Geozoic Era (Duration: about 60 million years up to present)	Atmosphere much clearer	Modern Plants Fruit Trees	Mammals Apes
. . . . about 25 million years ago				
VII	Present	Glaciation	Herbaceous Plants	Man

The future of man would continuously face colder glacial periods for approximately another
20 million years, before geological change brings to the surface of the earth a warmer climate.
In the meantime, man's civilization will face repeated glacial and interglacial periods. In the
former, civilization would become more reserved and in the latter it would prosper, as we are
experiencing now. After the age of man, new species would further develop as the climate
changes towards warmer in the far future.

Fig. 25   Biospirallic Development

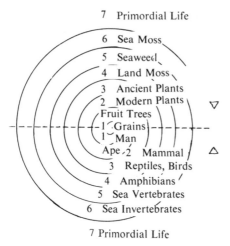

7   Primordial Life
6   Sea Moss
5   Seaweed
4   Land Moss
3   Ancient Plants
2   Modern Plants
Fruit Trees
1   Grains
1   Man
Ape 2   Mammal
3   Reptiles, Birds
4   Amphibians
5   Sea Vertebrates
6   Sea Invertebrates

7   Primordial Life

This chart shows another way to approach understanding historical development. At large, the entire period of biological development on the earth has taken over 3 billion years in accordance with geological and celestial change. This entire process generally orbits in seven stages, in a spirallic motion. The drawing shows a philosophical view—Yin, botanical development, and Yang, zoological evolution, as well as warmer climatic periods and cooler climatic periods. Man, who is the most yang central life, can take all domains of biological life as his food, and is a turning point towards dephysicalization and spiritualization—the outgoing course, from the spirallic inward process of a long biological development.

chapter 3

Dietary Principles for Man

> To practice macrobiotic order in the way of
> eating is the highest art man has ever produced.
> It is the way to achieve freedom and
> it is the way to practice freedom. Because
> of this, man can know life and death, and he
> shall know his eternal life.

> December, 1976

1. Standard Diet

As we see in biological development and in the nature of man within the universe, man and his environment are inseparable. When the environment changes, man changes, and he has to change, to maintain his existence. In order to change, he exercises his consciousness to choose and prepare the quality and volume of food suitable to his requirements within the changing environment. And in order to choose and prepare the proper food, man needs to have proper understanding of the law of nature, the order of the universe. Because he changes his body, mind, and spirit through the change of what he consumes, everyone is free for his own destiny, and is entirely responsible for his life. Man is always his own master, and there is no one else other than himself who is able to control him.

However, if he does not know how to change his body, mind, and spirit, man will not be able to adapt to the changing environment, and this would result in the eventual termination of his humanhood. Throughout the centuries there have been many philosophical, religious, and scientific recommendations to improve his human quality, and there have been many social and spiritual attempts through reformation or revolution to secure better living conditions. However, if such recommendations do not serve practically in the improvement of the quality of blood cells, as well as mental and spiritual qualities as a whole, through simple methods that everyone is able to practice, they are useless.

Traditional Dietary Teaching of the Jewish People
Since before the time of Abraham, the main food of the Jewish people has been wheat and other cereal grains. The teaching of Moses about dietary disciplines appears in the Old Testament, the Book of Leviticus. Unleavened bread and matzoh used for special occasions symbolize their main food.

Among some Orthodox Jewish people, Kosher practices are still maintained, in which grains, beans, and vegetables are the staple food, and special cooking is required for meat and animal food in order to avoid their harmful influences. Shellfish are also avoided because they can easily decay. Other fish, and fruits, are usually not prohibited.

In order to develop and maintain humanhood, its state of health, freedom and happiness—physical, mental, spiritual conditions as a whole—proper dietary practice is the most essential beyond any other measure. Without food, man as well as all life does not exist. From food, life has come as well as man. For this very reason, the ancestors of various traditional races have left to us teachings and sayings, customs and traditions, ceremonies and festivities which are revealing to us the essential importance of what we take as food.

Generally, in the temperate climate, where four seasons clearly alternate, and where the major civilizations and cultures of the world are prospering, the following way of eating should be standard, with necessary modifications, needless to say.

Principles:

1. Each meal should consist of food of vegetable quality, with occasional supplements of animal food if necessary.
2. The principal food in each meal, which should make up more than one-half the meal in volume, should be whole cereal grains and their products, including occasional supplements of legumes (beans).
3. Vegetables should be primarily cooked, with variations in cooking methods. Selection of vegetables should follow according to seasonal change. Vegetables grown locally are preferred to vegetables grown at a distance.
4. Sea vegetables can be used as additional vegetables in lesser quantity, and less frequently than land vegetables.
5. Fruits and nuts can be occasionally used as a supplement if they are grown in the same climate.
6. Animal food should be minor in volume and less than 15% of the whole meal, and eaten always together with vegetables.
7. Seasoning should be primarily with unrefined sea salt and vegetable quality oil. Tropical and semi-tropical spices, and aromatic herbs should be usually avoided.
8. Beverages should be made using herbs grown in the same climate.

One example of this standard diet is as follows:

Example of Standard Dietary Recommendations

1. In every meal, at least 50% or more in volume should be whole cereal grains, using a variety of cooking methods. Whole cereal grains are: brown rice, whole wheat, whole wheat bread, whole wheat chapati, whole wheat noodles, barley, millet, oats, oatmeal, rye, rye bread, corn, corn on the cob, corn grits, buckwheat groats, buckwheat noodles, etc.

Ise Shrine in Japan

The Grand Ise Shrine situated in Ise City, Mie Province. is the most central shrine in Japan. It is composed of two great shrines and other subsidiary shrines. The two are the Inner Shrine, NAIGU (内宮) and the Outer Shrine, GEGU (外宮). The internal shrine has been dedicated to the Heavenly Shining Great Spirit, AMA-TERASU-OOMIKAMI (天照大御神) symbolizing the sun and the radiating infinity. The external shrine is dedicated to the Great Grain Spirit, TOYO-UKE-NO-OOKAMI (豊受大神) symbolizing food and prosperity. The former is also representing heaven, while the latter represents the earth. Ise shrine has been a spiritual center of Japan for 2,000 years.

2.   Every day, 5% or so in volume (1 or 2 small bowls) of *miso*[1] soup or *tamari*[1] soy sauce soup. Taste should be mild. Contents should be various vegetables, sea-weeds, beans and grains; change frequently.

3.   About 20% to 30% in volume of each meal may be vegetables: 2/3 of them cooked in various styles, including sauteeing, steaming, boiling, baking; 1/3 of them eaten as raw salad or very simply, briefly cooked. A supplement of pickles in various styles is also desirable. Potatoes, including sweet potatoes and yams, tomatoes, eggplant, avocado and any other tropical-origin vegetable should be avoided. Asparagus, spinach, beets, zucchini squash and a few others among common vegetables may need to be avoided in some instances as long as you are in a non-tropical climate.

4.   10%–15% in volume of the daily meal—cooked beans and seaweed. Beans preferred for daily use are *azuki* beans, chickpeas, lentils, and black beans. Other beans are for more occasional use. Seaweeds such as *hijiki, kombu, wakame, nori,* dulse, agar-agar, and Irish moss can be used in a variety of cooking methods, and are to be usually seasoned with a moderate use of *tamari* soy sauce or sea salt.[2]

5.   A few times a week, if necessary, a small volume of whitemeat fish and seafood may be used in a variety of cooking methods. Also, a fruit dessert may be used a few times a week, provided the fruits are growing in the same climatic zone. Fruit juice is primarily not advisable to take often or in large quantity. Occasional use in hot weather may be enjoyed in small volume.

   Roasted seeds, roasted nuts, with slight salt taste, may be enjoyed as a snack or supplement as well as roasted grains and beans, and dried fruit.

6.   Beverage: roasted *bancha* twig tea; *Mu* tea, dandelion tea, burdock and dried root tea, and other non-aromatic herb teas, as well as cereal grain coffee or tea, are

---

[1] *Miso* is processed from soybeans and cereal grains such as barley, rice and wheat, with sea salt, for a period longer than 1–1/2 years, through slow fermentation. *Miso* is a paste form, and *tamari* soy sauce is a liquid form processed from similar ingredients. *Miso* and *tamari* have been used for many centuries in oriental countries in preparation of daily meals—*miso* for daily soup base and occasional sauces, and *tamari* soy sauce for a different soup base in the daily meal, and for seasoning of vegetables and other dishes. The word "tamari" indicates a very thick liquid squeezed from the fermented *miso*, but in macrobiotic use it is used to distinguish traditional, naturally-made soy sauce from soy sauce artificially made in a short time by commercial and chemical processes.

[2] *Sea Salt*: Since biological life had its origin in the primitive ocean, human blood and other body fluids contain salts including many varieties of minerals. Sodium chloride (NaCl)—pure salt—is not the only mineral compound which we need although it occupies the largest volume. Refined sea salt, which is nearly pure sodium chloride, is unsuitable to form our human blood and other body fluids. The traditional way of production of sea salt with natural sunshine and cleaning with water is the best available method. Sea salt for daily use should contain 8% to 12% other mineral compounds besides 88% to 92% NaCl. Taste and quality of dishes and pickles seasoned or processed with such unrefined sea salt is greatly different in richness, and nutritional value is much higher than with refined salt.

Mu Tea: There are two kinds of Mu tea available: one is mixed with nine different natural herbs, and one with 16. The formula of Mu tea was composed by George Ohsawa in 1963 from traditional oriental health herb teas. The effectiveness of this drink is to maintain the general vitality without unhealthy stimulation. This is a more yang beverage than other common drinks.

recommended for daily use, including any traditional tea which does not have an aromatic fragrant odor and stimulant effect.

7. Food categories generally excluded from the standard daily diet:
    —Mammals' meat, animal fat, poultry, dairy food.
    —Tropical, semi-tropical fruits and fruit juice, wine and other alcoholic beverages, soda, artificial drinks and beverages, coffee, dyed tea, all aromatic stimulant teas such as mint or peppermint tea.
    —Sugar, honey, all sorts of syrups, saccharine and other artificial sweeteners (rice honey, barley malt and any other sweeteners processed from grain or grain sprouts may be used in small volumes to add sweet taste if necessary).
    —All chemicalized food such as colored, preserved, sprayed, and chemically-treated foods. All refined, polished grains, flours and their products. Mass-produced industrialized food, including many canned and frozen foods.
    —Hot spices; any aromatic, stimulant foods, accessories, and beverages; artificial vinegar.

8. Additional advice:
    —The use of oil should be preferably such vegetable quality as cold-pressed sesame oil and corn oil, to be used in cooking in reasonable, moderate volume.
    —For condiments, the followings are to be normally used:
        1. *Gomashio*[3] or Sesame Salt (between 8 and 14 parts roasted sesame seeds with 1 part sea salt, mixed and partly crushed together). 10–12 parts seeds to 1 part salt are average.
        2. Roasted seaweed powder, such as kelp powder and *wakame* powder.
        3. *Umeboshi* plums[4]—salt-pickled plums.
        4. *Tekka*[5]—condiment processed from root vegetables and *miso*.
        5. *Tamari* soy sauce (moderate use, for seasoning).
    —Beverage: other than the above-mentioned natural beverages, hot water and water may be taken only when you are thirsty—but comfortably.
    —It is recommended to eat 2–3 times per day regularly, as much quantity as desired, provided the proportion is generally correct and chewing very well-preferably more than 50 times per mouthful. We should avoid eating for approximately three hours before sleeping.

---

[3] *Gomashio* (胡麻塩): "goma"=sesame seed, "shio"=salt.

[4] *Umeboshi Plum* (梅干): Plums pickled with sea salt for many months after drying are called *ume* (plum)—*boshi* (dry) in Japan. Usually, beefsteak plants are pickled together with the plums to add an appetizing red color and flavor. Oriental countries have been using them as frequently as every day. Appetite and digestion are stimulated by consuming half of one piece of *umeboshi* plum. They also aid in maintaining blood quality in a slight alkaline condition, according to oriental practice.

[5] *Tekka* (鉄火): The meaning of *tekka* is "iron fire"—from *tetsu* (鉄), iron, and *ka* (火), fire. This traditional condiment is made of carrot roots, burdock roots and lotus roots, finely chopped and sauteed together with sesame oil in addition to *miso*, for a long time, until it has the appearance of a black powder. The process is traditionally done in cast iron pans. Oriental countries use *tekka* widely as a condiment which is said to enrich the blood.

Recommendation of a standard diet is not limited to the above example. A few hundred varieties of meals can be created from the standard suggestions. Following the above general combinations of food varieties, similar combinations can be produced including variations of the percentage of food categories. Furthermore, meals should vary in volume, in quality, in preparation and in the manner of eating, depending upon change of environment, age, sex difference, traditional background, climate, and season, as well as social and personal need. The practice of intuitive judgment in those aspects is essentially important for everyone's health and happiness. Therefore, we need to apply the understanding of natural order in terms of a balance between antagonistic and complemental factors, yin and yang.

2. Yin and Yang in Daily Food

In the practice of daily diet covering a variety of foods, we need to exercise our proper selection of the kinds, quality and volume of both vegetable and animal food. In order to choose properly, we need to apply our intuitive and traditional native judgment which is much more practical than any scientific data and information, as mankind has practiced throughout hundreds of thousands of years.

With some minor exceptions, most vegetable-quality food is more yin than animal quality food, because of the following factors:

1. Vegetable species are fixed or stationary, growing in one place, while animal species are independently self-mobile, able to cover a larger space by their activity.

2. Vegetable species universally manifest their structure in an expanding growth form, the major growing portion manifesting the earth's expanding forces from the ground upwards towards the sky, or spreading over the ground laterally. On the other hand, animal species are generally forming compacted and separate unities. Vegetables have more expanded forms growing outwards such as branches and leaves, while animal bodies are formed in a more inwards direction with compacted organs and cells.

Fig. 26

Green Plant Cell   **Typical Animal Cell**

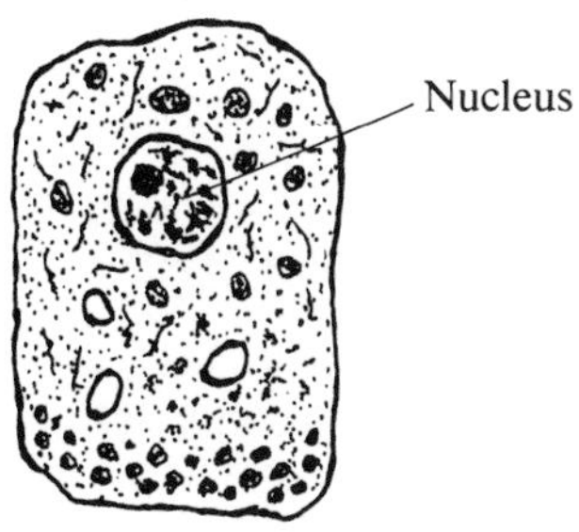

Nucleus

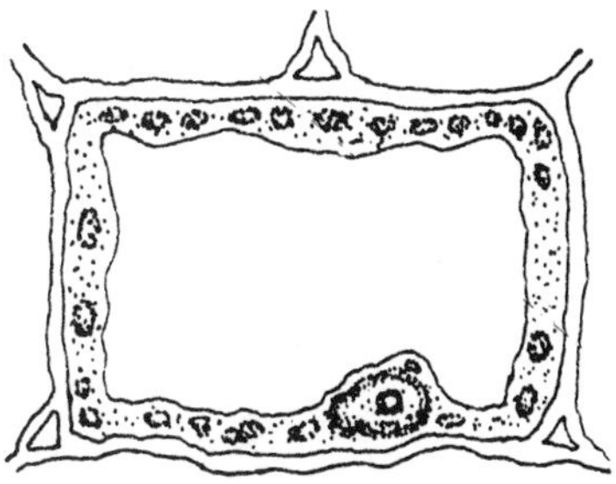

More expanded form—Yin   More contracted form—Yang

3. The body temperatures of plants are cooler than some species of animals and generally they inhale carbon dioxide (CO_2) and exhale oxygen (O_2).[6] Animal species are generally inhaling O_2 and exhaling CO_2. Vegetables are mainly represented by the color green, chlorophyll, while animals are manifested in the color red, hemoglobin. Their chemical structures resemble each other, yet their nuclei are respectively magnesium (Mg) in the case of chlorophyll, and iron (Fe) in the case of hemoglobin.

The nucleus of chlorophyll, magnesium, possibly transmutes into the nucleus of hemin, iron, by taking two oxygen.

Chlorophyll a (green)
(plants)

Hemin (red)
(animals)

$$Mg_{24}^{12} + 20_{16}^{8} \cdots (?)_{56}^{28} \cdots Fe_{56}^{26}$$

(?) is the transitory stage.

Although vegetable species are more yin than animal species and animals are more yang than vegetables, there are different degrees even among the same species and within one body. We can distinguish these differences of quality in accordance with the following standard of judgment:

As a general principle, when we use vegetable quality in the warmer season or region—more yang environment, it is safer to choose more yin quality of vegetables, and when we use them in the colder season or region, more yang quality of vegetables. If we are in the temperate zone, more yin vegetables should be cooked a longer time with the possible addition of other yang factors including heat, pressure,

---

[6] O_2 vs. CO_2: Among all elements, some elements are more yin than others and some are more yang than others, according to their size, mass weight, freezing and boiling points, chemical and thermal reactions, as well as spectroscopic color and other characteristics. In the examination of these factors, among the first eight light elements, oxygen and carbon show an antagonistic and complemental relation, with oxygen—yin, and carbon—yang. Accordingly, the carbon and oxygen relation works as a major force in the balance and harmony of nature. From the above view, O_2 is yin and CO_2 yang, which work in balance in the biological world. Animals who take in yin O_2 and expel yang CO_2 are more yang, and vegetables, which take in CO_2 and expel O_2 are more yin. (Yin attracts yang, yang attracts yin; yin repels yin, yang repels yang.)

Yin and Yang in the Vegetable Kingdom

	Yin (▽) Centrifugal	Yang (△) Centripetal
Environment:	Warmer, more tropical	Colder, more polar
Season:	Grows more in spring and summer	Grows more in autumn and winter
Soil:	More watery and sedimentary	More dry and volcanic
Growing direction:	Vertically growing upwards; expanding horizontally underground	Vertically growing downward expanding horizontally above the ground
Growing speed:	Growing faster	Growing slower
Size:	Larger, more expanded	Smaller, more compacted
Height:	Taller	Shorter
Texture:	Softer	Harder
Water content:	More juicy and watery	More dry
Color:	Purple—blue—green—yellow—brown—orange—red	
Odor:	Stronger smell	Less smell
Taste:	Spicy—sour—sweet—salty—bitter	
Chemical components:	More K and other yin elements	Less K and other yin elements
Nutritional components:	Fat—protein—carbohydrate—mineral	
Cooking time:	Faster cooking	Slower cooking

Fig. 27   The Opposite Characteristics—Yin and Yang —of Plants and the Human Body

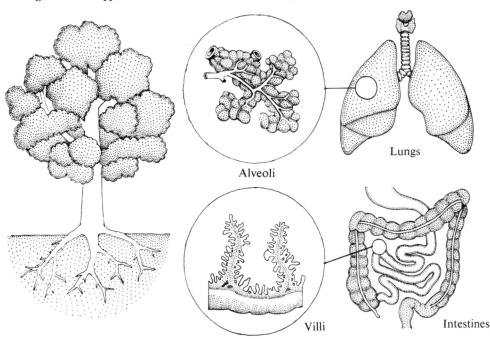

Alveoli

Lungs

Villi

Intestines

The leaves of the tree—expanded structures—breathe in CO_2 and give out O_2, while human lungs —compacted structures—breathe in O_2 and give out CO_2. Roots absorb liquid nourishment from the soil in the case of plants, while in the case of human beings, intestinal villi, which have an inverse structure, absorb the nourishment of food molecules. Many other opposite characteristics can be observed in the structures and functions of plants and the human body.

and salt, and more yang vegetables can be less cooked. In general, yinner vegetables give more physical, mental effects for expansion and slowing down metabolism as well as cooling body temperature, while more yang quality cooked vegetables give us the effects of contraction, activating metabolism and increasing body temperature, although some very yin vegetable quality foods such as spices, aromatic stimulant plants and drinks can give a temporary activation of metabolism and higher body temperature, and very yang vegetables such as root vegetables cooked with salt seasoning can give us a temporary slowing of metabolism.

Yin and Yang in the Animal Kingdom

	Yin (▽) Centrifugal	Yang (△) Centripetal
Environment:	Warmer and more tropical; also, in warm current	Colder and more polar; also in cold current.
Air humidity:	More humid	More dry
Species:	Generally more ancient	Generally more modern
Size:	Larger, more expanded	Smaller, more compacted
Activity:	Slower moving and more inactive	Faster moving and more active
Body temperature:	Colder	Warmer
Texture:	Softer, more watery and oily	Harder and drier
Color of flesh:	Transparent—white—brown—pink—red—black	
Odor:	More odor	Less odor
Taste:	Putrid—sour—sweet—salty—bitter	
Chemical components:	Less sodium (Na) and other yang elements	More sodium (Na) and other yang elements
Nutritional components:	Fat . . . . Protein . . . . Minerals	
Cooking time:	Shorter	Longer

In general practice, when we use animal quality it is preferable to choose more yin quality foods, and it is safer to use them together with vegetables to harmonize each other. As mentioned before, more primitive species are more recommendable than modern species.

In the temperate zone, vegetable quality food should be the majority and animal quality the minority in volume, as we saw in the previous chapter. However, in both categories of food, each plant or animal body has its own balance: of carbohydrate, protein, fat, minerals and vitamins in the case of vegetables, and of protein, fat, and minerals in the case of animal food. It is therefore advisable to consume a whole plant or whole body of either species. For example, carrot roots with their green tops; dandelion roots and their leaves; and in the case of animal food, smaller fish can be eaten whole, including head, bones and tail. The exception to this principle is grains and fruits, because they have an independent unity separate from the other parts of the plant.

In consideration of yin and yang in various kinds of food, we are able to classify, from yin to yang or from yang to yin, the entire scope of food as well as within each category of food. For example, among the food arrangement recommended in the standard diet in the temperate climate, we can see the following examples:

Celery, for example, grows in the warm season or climate; grows quickly; is long in shape; is fragile and watery; has a strong smell and taste; cooks quickly; and is pale green in color. We can easily see that celery has many yin characteristics. For another example, a *carrot* is more hard and compact, takes a longer time to grow and continues growing in the cool season; is orange in color with a mild taste and odor; is a more dry vegetable; takes a longer time to cook. Among vegetables, then, we may classify a carrot as more yang. As for a grain of *wheat*, it is very small and

General Yin (▽) and Yang (△) Categorization of Food

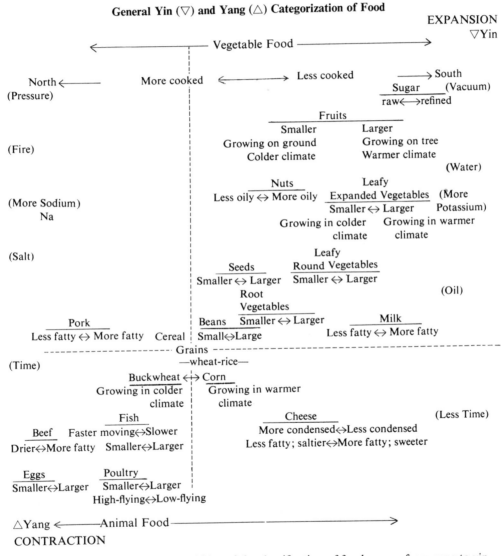

EXPANSION
▽Yin

The above chart gives the general idea of the classification of food groups from yang to yin, from yin to yang. However, more precise classification should be made upon examination of environmental conditions, nature and structure, chemical compounds, and effect upon our physical and mental conditions. Also, cooking can greatly change food qualities from yin to yang and yang to yin.

compact, and may grow in cool climates and cool season; matures slowly; is more dry and hard, and brown in color, with very subtle odor and taste; a high carbohydrate content and a need for longer cooking time. We may see that *wheat* as well as other grains are relatively more yang in comparison with many other kinds of vegetable food. Among fish, the *shrimp* is small, red or pink, fast moving, and contains plenty of minerals and less fat; this places it on the more yang side of the seafood kingdom. On the other hand, a *carp* is large, soft, fat, slow moving, and lives in warm currents—all yin factors. *Brook trout* live in cold streams, move quickly, are more hard and compact with less fat—so we may see that they are more yang fish than the carp. Using the same criteria, we may develop the ability to judge the yin and yang qualities of all different kinds of food.

3. Environmental Modifications and Personal Adjustment

Although the recommendation of the standard arrangement of food in the temperate climate is workable universally for those who are living a normal life, we should consider some adjustments and modifications according to the change of environmental conditions and personal requirements. Considerations of these adjustments are mainly dealing with the following respects: (1) tradition; (2) climate; (3) seasonal change; (4) geographical conditions; (5) social conditions; (6) personal variations, including sex and age differences and variations in activity; and others.

A. The Traditional Way of Eating

Generally speaking, if we continue to live in a certain place throughout our lifetime or a large part of our life, we should follow the dietary practices which have been traditionally exercised by the majority of people in that particular place. Like most traditional villages and towns throughout the world, the people of Hunza, the people of Bhutan, or the Eskimos, who have maintained certain patterns of eating, have been able to keep their lives in healthy condition; but if they change their way of eating into a foreign custom such as the use of modern manufactured

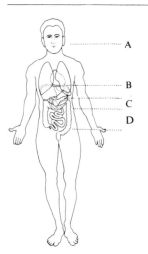

Alternative Digestive Processes, Yin ($\triangledown$) and Yang ($\triangle$)

A. *Saliva*—Saliva is an alkaline liquid ($\triangle$), mainly digesting and decomposing carbohydrates.
B. *Stomach Juice*—Gastric juice is acid ($\triangledown$), digesting and decomposing mainly fat and protein.
C. *Liver and Gall Bladder Bile and Pancreatic Juice*—These digestive liquids are alkaline ($\triangle$), mainly decomposing fat, protein, and carbohydrate.
D. *Intestinal Juice*—This juice is acid ($\triangledown$), digesting and decomposing all carbohydrate, protein and fat. These decomposed food molecules turn into the bloodstream after absorption, which is weak alkaline ($\triangle$).

food, they inevitably lose their adaptability to their environment and they would start to disappear as we are seeing in many cases.

The traditional way of eating has been developed through many centuries by the accumulation of numerous experiences from generation to generation. In many parts of the world they even developed religious and ceremonial customs dedicated to certain kinds of food which their ancestors experienced through the long period of history as the most valuable food in their specific environment. Shintoism in Japan enshrines the spirit of rice and other grains. North and South American Indians have a mythology of gods relating to maize. Jewish ancestors respected unleavened bread as a holy means to be together with God. Greeks and Romans worshipped gods of grains. Numerous other examples in ancient times are handed down to their offspring who would continue to live in that environment, teaching them about the way of eating. In many cases, such tradition includes special types of dishes and special types of cooking. Proverbs and parables are also left by them to tell the importance of certain ways of eating in that environment. Therefore, wherever we go and live we should respect and practice the way of eating traditionally developed in that locality over many centuries. From such traditional ways of eating, traditional cultures have been developed and kept. To practice the traditional way of eating is to respect traditional culture.

B. Modification According to Climate

The world climate is generally divided into five climatic regions in terms of the way of eating: polar, cool, temperate, semi-tropical, and tropical. The polar climate generally gives a colder atmosphere throughout the year. The cool climate generally gives a long colder season and a short warm season. The temperate climate gives generally four different seasons. The semi-tropical climate gives a longer period of warm weather and a shorter period of cool weather, and the tropical climate gives a more hot climate throughout the year. When we live in different climates, our way of eating should be different.

Under the colder atmosphere (yin), we should adapt ourselves to the environment by making our food of more yang quality, applying heavier cooking and even using animal quality to some degree. People who have been living in Mongolia and Northern Manchuria, despite the fact that most Asians have been using more grains and vegetables, have developed their strength by eating heavily cooked food and by including animal food in their diet. Similarly, people in Scandinavia have used fish

---

How to Minimize the Poisonous Effects of Animal Food
For meat—soaking in salt water before cooking, and when eating, treat with salt and a small volume of hot spices. Leafy vegetables should accompany meat at all times.
For poultry—vegetable quality of oil and unrefined sea salt.
For shellfish such as lobster, crabmeat, clams and oysters—horseradish, grated and raw.
For fishes living near the seashore—onions, scallions cooked and uncooked.
For fishes living a little farther out to sea—radish and long radish (*daikon*), grated and raw.
For fishes living still farther out to sea—ginger, grated and raw.
For fishes in the far distant and deep sea—green mustard.
These treatments and accessories for those particular foods have been traditionally practiced, from long experience in various countries, as dietary custom.

and seafood in their daily diet. On the other hand, people who live in India, in the overwhelming majority, exclude the consumption of meat and eggs, and apply lighter cooking than the people who are living in China. People in Africa have been traditionally depending on rice, tapioca and bananas and have not been using heavy animal food. People who live in Southern California cannot tolerate the dietary practices of New England for a long period, unless they change their cooking methods, including lighter cooking and the addition of some raw vegetables and occasional use of fruits.

People who live in the higher mountains have eaten differently from people who live in the lower plains. People who live in the inland section of continents naturally differ their way of eating from the people who live on the seashore along the ocean. Even though it has been the tradition that the principal food has been grain for the major populations of the world, those who are in colder Eastern Europe, such as Russia, eat more buckwheat (more yang), those who are in Southwestern Europe, such as Spain and Portugal, eat more rice and wheat, and those who are in Central America eat more corn and beans (more yin) to adapt to their climate.

In the polar region, our food should be grains, land and sea vegetables, fish, meat and food processed from them. Grains should be more buckwheat, northern millet, and northern winter wheat. Vegetables are to be treated with heavier cooking by more fire, pressure, salt and time. Fish and meat should be treated in the traditional way in such regions, and may well consist of the larger portion of the meal than vegetable-quality food in some occasions.

In the cool region, our food should be grains, beans, land and sea vegetables, fish, seafood and other animal quality as well as a minor quantity of fruits growing in such climates. Grains are to be more wheat, oats, barley, rye, millet, buckwheat, and a northern short grain variety of rice. Vegetables are to be chosen in that climate and generally well-cooked, except during the warm summer season. Animal food is to be prepared according to the traditional way of cooking in such places. The portion of animal food should be far less than vegetable quality, though it may be consumed frequently.

In the temperate region, our food should be grains, beans, land and sea vegetables, smaller portions or infrequent use of animal food, and a small volume of fruits and food processed from them. Grains and beans as well as vegetables can be chosen from the various kinds growing in the same climate. Fruits should also be chosen in the same climate, according to growing season. The cooking should be adjusted according to season, moderately applying fire, pressure, salt and oil with any other basic seasonings.

In the semi-tropical region, food should be grains, beans, land and sea vegetables, a small volume of fruits and very infrequent use of animal food, and food processed from these things. All of these products should be chosen in the same climatic region: for example, medium or long grain rice, summer wheat, and middle sized beans. The cooking should be applying fire, salt, and water moderately with other basic seasonings. A portion of vegetables may be raw in the form of salad or pickles.

In the tropical region, our food should be grains, beans, land and sea vegetables, and more fruits than in any other region, as well as food processed from them; almost no animal food. The cooking should be much lighter, and oil and spices may

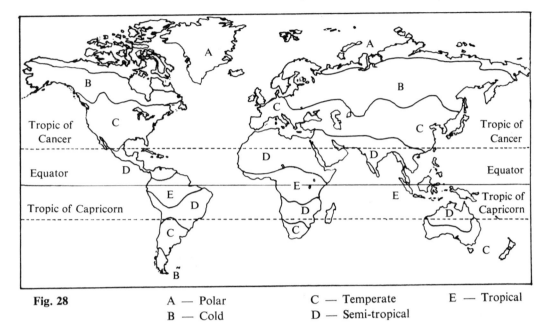

Fig. 28

A — Polar	C — Temperate	E — Tropical
B — Cold	D — Semi-tropical	

be used in a larger volume than in any other region.

C. Adjustment According to Seasonal Change

In most parts of the world we experience the change of seasons, colder to warmer, warmer to colder. In the temperate region we experience this change most clearly in the alternating four seasons of spring, summer, autumn and winter. On the other hand, the polar and tropical regions do not experience the clear change of seasons. The majority of the world's people are living in areas where seasonal change is experienced. Natural biological life—plants and animals—change their species' qualities and numbers according to the change of season. Man also should follow this seasonal change. If we eat summer products such as melon and summer squash in the winter season, we lose our adaptability to the immediate environment. The development of modern transporation has been violating this seasonal order by , importing food from regions of different climates.

Each season and each month, spring to autumn, nature produces certain kinds of grains, beans, vegetables, and fruits. These products should be consumed in that particular season or month and products growing in different seasons or months should be avoided. During the winter season, which does not produce natural vegetation as much as other seasons, we should consume such foods that are storable by simple methods. Grains, beans, seeds, root vegetables and many hard leafy vegetables as well as some autumn fruits can be stored very easily and therefore can be used throughout the winter. With the exception of food stored by traditional methods, including pickling, drying, and smoking, food preserved by canning, freezing and other artificial and chemical methods should be avoided.

D. Adjustment According to Geographical Conditions

Although the same pattern of food is generally applicable to people living in the same climatic region, people who live in a mountainous region should arrange their food depending upon their particular locality. A mountain does not produce many plants usually found growing in the plain, but instead produces different varieties. For example, in the case of grains, the mountainous area in the temperate region produces buckwheat and millet, and seldom wheat and rice. Those who live in such a place should eat those grains growing in their area and should not trade with the villages on the plain for wheat and rice.

Similarly, people who live on the island or seashore near the ocean are living in more mineral-containing air. Vegetation in such areas is also more enriched with certain minerals. By eating them, people become able to adapt to their environment. On the other hand, people living deep inland on large continents should consume plants growing in their area. The traditional practice of such eating together with the influence of environmental conditions has made people who are living on islands or at the seashore, smaller than the people who are living in the inland areas of continents.

In the same way, people who are living in drier air should differ their way of eating from the people who live in high-humidity areas, with the consumption of more liquid. The major part of Western Europe where it is less humid than in the Far Eastern islands (such as Japan, Formosa, and the Philippines) have traditionally used a smaller volume of salt, and a major part of North America which is much drier than Europe, uses more water and beverages, salad and fruits than the people in Western Europe.[7]

E.   Modification According to Social Conditions

Primitive societies, in comparison with civilized societies, are maintaining a much more traditional way of eating. Undeveloped countries have a more natural method of cultivation and preparation of food. Food quality as well as all related problems of eating is often more health-producing in primitive societies than in civilized countries. People who live in highly civilized societies are no longer consuming the quality of food that their ancestors have been eating for many centuries. Similarly, people living in towns are eating a more artificial quality of food in comparison with people living in the country. Their whole lives are depending upon unnatural, mass-produced commercialized food. Similarly, in the organized communities such as schools, hospitals, the military, and business establishments, people's blood is totally artificialized by commercially catered food services. Those who live in the civilized society, especially within towns and community establishments, should be more

---

[7] Stories of giants are always related with continents, while stories of midgets come from islands. For example: the Leprechauns of Ireland; the Kappa of Japan; King Kong and Paul Bunyan from the American continent, and the Abominable Snowman from the Himalayas. Peninsular parts of continents have mixed stories, such as the German and English fairy tales which include both giants and little people. People living in large continents have the tendency to appreciate large structures, while people living on islands appreciate more minutely refined arts. Continent—space larger—yin; island—space smaller—yang.

Mt. Kilimanjaro is located in a tropical region, but from the foot to the top, scenery of all different climatic regions can be seen: tropical, semi-tropical, temperate, cool, and polar. People who are living on a mountain should adjust their way of eating according to the difference of altitude as if they were living in a different climatic region.

cautious to choose natural quality of food and to practice slightly lighter cooking than in undeveloped areas.

F. *Personal Variations*

Even if we live in the same climatic region at the same time and same place, every person has a different constitution, activity, and occupation together with the difference of sex and age. Those who are engaged in more mental activity should consume a slightly more yin quality of food, and those who are engaged in a more physical occupation should eat a slightly more yang quality. The former can take less quantity of food and liquid, while the latter may consume a larger volume of food and drink.

Man, according to his biological constitution and his comparatively wider social activities, may eat more variety of food including a small volume of animal food, except in the tropical region. On the other hand, woman, in her biological nature, may consume a smaller volume of food, and almost exclusively of vegetable quality. Accordingly, man may take slightly more minerals and salt in his food, while woman should take slightly less.

During the growing age, our food should be slightly more yin—more volume in proportion to the body size, especially in protein and carbohydrate, more volume of liquid and more frequent use of natural sweets, as well as less use of salt. As we reach the adult age, the volume of food should become proportionally smaller, and as we reach the older age, it should become further smaller. Animal food should also become successively less in volume, and when we reach the older age—about

---

Primitive and Modern Food and the Problem of Health

"The studies of Price in these islands are particularly important. He found that on the more isolated islands, where the diet was still basically oat products and sea food, the people maintained fine physiques and high immunity to dental caries. The percentage of decay ranged from 0.7 to 1.3 per cent, meaning that an average of one in each hundred teeth was affected. As the natives used the smoke-permeated thatch, which would be removed from their homes at intervals, for fertilizer, this was tested by Price for the growing of oats, and it was found more than to double the rate of growth. The natives claimed similar results, and we may expect that the fertilizer added to the nutritional qualities of the food as well.

"On some of the islands, Price found modern foods—white flour products, canned marmalades, canned vegetables, sweetened fruit juices, chocolate and confections of all types—to be in widespread use. Here the condition of health was markedly lower than elsewhere. Dental decay among children averaged as high as 32.4 per cent in one area, and was generally widespread everywhere. In the port of Stornoway on the Isle of Lewis, twenty-five of a group of a hundred young adults were found wearing artificial restorations. In the same place a sanatorium had been erected to care for the increasing number of patients afflicted with tuberculosis, a disease that is virtually unknown on the more isolated islands where native foods are yet in use.

"The general dietary experiences in Europe are significant in the study of different modes of human nutrition. We find that the few racial groups who, during the past century, have maintained or re-established sufficient phases of the native dietary customs have uniformly had various kinds of physical immunity not found elsewhere. Throughout the greater part of the continent, where modern foods are in general use, there are many signs of human degeneration. This is in the form of poor physical development, low resistance to all forms of disease, and dental decay so serious that half the adult population in some areas wear artificial restorations." (Excerpts from *Primitive Man and His Food*—Chapter 4, "Dietary Habits in Europe," by Arnold De Vries, pp. 42–43.)

the early sixties in man, and the middle fifties in woman—food should become almost exclusively vegetable quality in the temperate and warmer climatic regions. For example, protein may be supplied from the products of whole grains and beans. At the same time, the intake of salts should become gradually less during old age, and fruits and sweets as well.

Knowing the order of the universe, yin and yang, we follow the changing conditions of our environment by changing what we eat. At the same time, using the understanding of yin and yang, we modify our physical and mental conditions by adjusting our food. When we are thus able to manage freely what we consume as our daily food, we are exercising freedom in our life. The principle of exercising our freedom to manage our biological and psychological, social and spiritual orientation is nothing but harmonizing ourselves to the environment.

1. In the more yin environment we make ourselves more yang.
    In the more yang environment we make ourselves more yin.
2. To make ourselves more yang, we take more yang.
    To make ourselves more yin, we take more yin.

Health is the state of freely managing the balance between yin and yang.

4. Principles of Cooking

No other animal species developed on this earth for over three billion years has learned the art of cooking, as man is applying in his daily diet. As a result of his intellectual development which has been advanced by the eating of cereal grains over millions of years, man started to use fire during the period of the ice age in order to adapt to his environment. Fire gives energy, vitalizing the physical, mental and spiritual activities. For this very reason, man began to build his culture and civilization.

In the beginning, fire was applied to his food. Then, it was applied to produce his clothing; and further, to build his dwelling, together with producing tools and equipment out of the natural materials surrounding him. Because of fire absorbed into his body in the form of food, and because of fire surrounding him in the form of culture, man's emotional, intellectual, social, and ideological consciousness has rapidly grown. Man has become a completely different species from all other biological life on this earth. Prometheus made man free from his environment so that he

---

Yin and Yang in Human Activity

A yin type of activity is more mental, emotional, intellectual and philosophical work such as the arts, music, architecture, designing, accounting, legal work, administrative work, religious and spiritual activities, teaching, secretarial work, writing, planning and thinking.

Yang activities are more active physically and socially, including labor, construction, driving, distribution and selling, promotion, speaking, production, politics, martial arts, sports, dance, farming.

Yin types of activity and those who are engaged in such activities are nourished by more yin types of foods (their faces are generally longer), while yang types of activity and people who are engaged in such activities are resulting from a consumption of more yang types of foods (their faces are generally more round or square).

is no longer subservient to it, but has become able to adapt positively to manage his own destiny.

However, as he applies the use of fire in various domains of his life, resulting in a technological society, man has started to lose his ability to manage fire in the flexible adaptation to the natural environment, and he has become enslaved by the artificial fire environment which has grown beyond his control. Fire civilization, especially over the recent several thousand years, has been going on without proper guidance based upon the understanding of life and the order of the universe.

Internally, modern man is now suffering various physical and mental diseases through artificial and unnatural food and drink, and breathing polluted air, which have all been produced by the use of fire, and externally he is suffering various social conflicts and struggles, wars and battles which have resulted from the application of fire. The present current of human degeneration, physical and mental, social and spiritual, which is now developing to the extent of the possible extinction of homo sapiens, began originally in the improper use of fire, particularly in the preparation of food, which is the source of man's suitability to the earth.

Therefore, it is urgent and essential that everyone should understand the principles of cooking, to be applied in daily food. Such principles are not only to be applied to secure man's continuous existence as a human species, but also to be applied towards the further development of the quality of humanity, as the highest art man has ever produced. However great masterpieces there may be, including the work of Michelangelo and Leonardo da Vinci, Beethoven and Mozart as well as many others, they all are unable to create and change human life itself—except the art of cooking applied to our daily life.

The purpose of the art of cooking is to manage a part of the environment—minerals, water, biological life, atmosphere, pressure, and time—to become the simplest dishes in the most practically and delicately condensed form suitable for the smoothest transformation into a healthy, happy, free man.

Such principles contain the following aspects:

1. All food materials should be chosen from natural organic products growing in the same climatic region and in the same season.
2. All of these food materials should represent all stages of the entire biological development—mainly vegetable species in the case of normal adults not living in the polar region.
3. Such food materials should be alive until the beginning of cooking, and should be used in whole.
4. Cooking should center around whole grains and the first and second supplementary foods, land and sea vegetables. More ancient species should be cooked more; more recent species can be cooked less.
5. Before applying fire and water, chopped food materials should be placed separately—not mixed—to avoid interchange of quality.
6. When cutting food materials, it is preferable that each piece should represent both yin and yang qualities.
7. During the cooking process, we should refrain from frequent mixing and stirring and should, as much as possible, simply allow foods to mix themselves

during the natural process of cooking.

8. Excessive use of fire, water, pressure and time as well as the excessive use of salt, oil and any other seasoning, should be avoided.

9. Seasoning should be with natural quality products such as unrefined sea salt, cold-pressed vegetable oil, natural grain sweetener, and whole grain vinegar, and should be used moderately. The taste of the seasoning should not be evident, but should only be used to bring out and enhance the natural taste of the food itself, which should be the predominant taste.

10. The same style of cooking, same type of dish should not be repeated for a long period. It is preferable to change the style of cooking often, in order to adapt to the changing environment.

11. The best quality of fire to use for cooking is wood fire; next, charcoal; next, coal; followed by gas. Electric and microwave cooking are preferably avoided.

12. The best quality of water is good-quality well and spring water or mountain stream water. City water which is heavily chemicalized is not to be preferred, as well as distilled water.

13. Besides basic seasoning, various fragrant hot spices should be avoided or minimized, according to the climate.

14. Dishes should be arranged beautifully with the natural color of food, and conveniently for the order of eating. These dishes should be served gracefully and consumed with appreciation.

15. The atmosphere of the cooking and eating place should be kept clean and quiet, and those who cook, serve and eat should maintain a peaceful mind.

Even though we use the same quality of food material and the same place of cooking, with the same cooking utensils, the result of cooking and therefore the quality of each dish, comes out differently each time we cook. This depends largely upon our changing conditions, physical and mental, and for this very reason we are creating either the improvement or deterioration of our health. Those who cook, therefore, are required to be of the best health and understanding of yin and yang, the order of nature and the universe, together with a profound technique in the art of cooking. Such a person is apparently most valuable in human society, and because of him or her, a household, a community will become healthier and happier. Traditionally throughout history, women have been engaged in this most important role for humanity, and it is most essential that proper cooking is restored as soon as

---

Food and Fertility

Infertility is often due to wrong dietary practice. Heavy consumption of meat, eggs, and dairy food as well as sugar, soft drinks, and hot spices, causes disorders in the sexual organs and functions. Menstrual cramps can easily be eliminated by eliminating all animal food. Infertility is caused mostly by fat and mucus accumulation within the ovarian area and Fallopian tubes. Eating vegetable quality food according to macrobiotic principles restores the ability to conceive in such cases.

"An angel of the Lord appeared to the woman and said to her, "Though you are barren and have had no children, yet you will conceive and bear a son. Now, then, be careful not to take wine or strong drink and to eat nothing unclean."

("nothing unclean"=no animal food.)

The Old Testament, Judges, Ch. 13, 3–5.

possible in every family, in every community and in every country for the benefit of entire mankind.

5. Modern Considerations

The macrobiotic way of eating is based upon everyone's native common sense with the intuitive understanding of the relation between man and his environment. It is also managed by the sense of balance and harmony dynamically achieved between antagonistic and complementary factors, yin and yang. The macrobiotic way has been tested and experienced by hundreds of billions of people over hundreds of centuries, in most parts of the world, whether or not such practice was called "macrobiotics." On the other hand, scientific studies on food and nutrition in the modern age have commenced only within the past two centuries. These modern studies are still immature and imperfect in many respects, and would never reach a stage of perfection as long as they are using analytical methods almost exclusively and overlooking the dynamic relation of life and environment as an organic whole.

However, there are several problems to be understood from the view of modern science in connection with the macrobiotic way of eating in order to have clear and practical knowledge:

A.   The problem of calories

The present recommendation of calories being made by public institutions tends to overestimate the volume of calories required for the average person. The modern method of calculating the required calories for various activities indicates the calories discharged by such activities (which results from the volume and quality of food eaten), but does not indicate the calories really required for such activities. Therefore, recommendations based upon such examinations result in a progressively increasing recommendation of caloric intake in prosperous countries, where people are eating more enriched food, and a lower recommendation in countries where the people are eating more simply.

According to the macrobiotic view, one's natural appetite for natural-quality food properly prepared, and one's bowel movement occurring regularly once a day, are more practical barometers for determining the necessary volume of food as well as required calories. Caloric requirements vary generally between 1,200 and 1,800 daily depending upon personal need, if the standard diet is generally practiced in

---

Allergy with Cereal Grains and Flour

There are some occasions in which people develop allergic conditions from the consumption of cereal grains such as wheat and millet, and cereal flour products such as bread and noodles. People with such reactions have usually been consuming, especially from childhood, milk and other dairy food as well as sugar and sugar products consistently. There are many occasions among psychologically disturbed people who are unable to consume cereal grain products because of allergy. In such cases, it is recommended that consumption of larger volume of various cooked and uncooked vegetables together with beans and bean products should be encouraged along with the gradual reduction of animal food, dairy food, and sugar products. After a period of such change, it usually becomes possible to consume cereal grains and their products.

the temperate region with two to three meals per day. Furthermore, we have to consider that some foods convert into calories with higher speed than other foods. For example sugar processed from sugar cane produces calories rapidly, but the caloric discharge soon ceases; while glucose contained in cereal grains is slowly burning into calories and lasting longer. In this respect, a diet centered around grain and vegetables is far superior to a diet centered around meat and sugar.

B. *The problem of carbohydrates*

Carbohydrates are generally known as sugars, but in speaking of sugar we should specify the variety. There are generally four different types of sugar: glucose, fructose, lactose, and sucrose. They are common respectively in grains and vegetables in the case of glucose, in fruits in the case of fructose, in milk products in the case of lactose, and in sugar cane and beets in the case of sucrose.

For our physical activity, we need carbohydrate in our daily food in the form of glucose, especially polysaccharide glucose (complex sugar), and through its gradual decomposition our metabolism and activity is sustained. When we store excessive sugar within our organs such as the liver, it is stored in the form of polysaccharide glucose. On the other hand, other sugars—the sugar of fruits, milk, and cane or beets—give undesirable effects to our physical and mental condition, and produce numerous kinds of disease and abnormal symptoms, including schizophrenia, heart disease, diabetes, obesity, and many others. In order to cure those sicknesses, it is recommended to terminate or minimize the intake of such sugars but it is also important to replace such sugars with polysaccharides and continue to eat carbohydrates in this form.

Current Recommendation of Calories (Energy) in the United States

(Designed for the maintenance of good nutrition of practically all healthy people in the U.S.A.)

	Age (years)	Weight (kg.)	Weight (lbs.)	Height (cm.)	Height (in.)	Energy (kcal.)
Infants	0.0–0.5	6	14	60	24	kg x 117
	0.5–1.0	9	20	71	28	kg x 108
Children	1–3	13	28	86	34	1,300
	4–6	20	44	110	44	1,800
	7–10	30	66	135	54	2,400
Males	11–14	44	97	158	63	2,800
	15–18	61	134	172	69	3,000
	19–22	67	147	172	69	3,000
	23–50	70	154	172	69	2,700
	51+	70	154	172	69	2,700
Females	11–14	44	97	155	62	2,400
	15–18	54	119	162	65	2,100
	19–22	58	128	162	65	2,100
	23–50	58	128	162	65	2,000
	51+	58	128	162	65	1,800
Pregnant						+300
Lactating						+500

Prepared by Food and Nutrition Board, National Academy of Sciences—National Research Council, 1974.

Polysaccharide glucose is universally available in grains, beans, and many other common vegetables, and the macrobiotic diet is featuring the supply of carbohydrates in this form in the daily diet.

C.   *The problem of protein*

Recent trends in nutritional advice tend to overemphasize protein. It is true that the human body consists of protein in large part. However, (1) all protein required in our body does not necessarily come from protein itself, but there is a constant interchange between protein, carbohydrate and fat within our body; and (2) food is used not only for the formation of the body but also for the energy of daily activities. The ratio of food used for body construction to food used for activity should be, on the average, 1:7. Generally, protein is used for body construction and carbohydrates for the energy of activity, though they are somewhat interchangeable; and therefore carbohydrates are much more required in volume than protein in any circumstance, as long as physical metabolism is continuing.

In the macrobiotic way of eating, protein can be supplied from whole cereal grains, various beans and their products, and the occasional use of animal food. These proteins and their composition of amino acids including the balance of the eight essential amino acids are not inferior at all to proteins in meat, cheese, eggs, and other animal food. Probably the most ideally balanced amino acid suitable for man is the protein in brown rice. Vegetable protein is more flexible than animal protein in the ability of interchange between body construction and body energy for activity.

D.   *The problem of fat*

In modern prosperous societies, the consumption of fat is often larger than in other countries where people are eating whole grains as the principal food. Excessive volumes of carbohydrates and protein taken into the body tend to be stored in the form of fat at various locations in the body. Since fat is more yin than carbohydrates and protein, it has a tendency to be stored around the more yang, com-

---

Protein Content in Some Vegetable and Animal Foods (per 100 grams, unit gram)

Whole cereal grains:		Seeds and Nuts:	
Brown rice, various	7.4– 7.5	Various	11.0–29.7
Wheat, various	9.4–14.0	Meat and Poultry:	
Oats	13.0	Beef, various	13.6–21.8
Barley, various	8.2– 8.9	Pork, various	9.1–21.5
Rye, various	12.1–12.7	Chicken, various	14.5–23.4
Millet, various	9.9–12.7	Other birds and poultry	18.5–25.3
Buckwheat, various	11.0–14.5	Eggs, various	12.9–13.9
Corn, maize, various	8.2– 8.9	Dairy Food:	
Sorghum	11.0–12.7	Cheeses, various	13.6–27.5
Beans:		Sea Animals:	
Azuki beans	21.5	Fishes, various	16.4–25.4
Kidney beans	20.2	Shellfish	10.6–24.8
Peas, dried, various	21.7–24.1	Seafoods	15.0–20.0
Broad beans, various	25.1–26.0		
Soybeans, various	34.1–34.3		
Mung beans, various	23.0–24.2	*Source:* U.S. Department of Agriculture and	
Lima beans	20.4	Japan Nutritionist Association	

pacted organs such as the liver or kidneys, or the more yang active organs such as the heart.

The requirement of fat is much less than the common practice of fat intake in modern society, if the proportional balance between carbohydrate and protein is maintained in daily food. Because fat is convertible into the role of carbohydrate —a source of energy, and protein—a source of body construction, fat is more required in a diet which is unbalanced. For this reason, those who are not using whole grains as a principal food need more fat intake in their daily diet. However, when they take fat in the form of animal fat such as meat fat, poultry, eggs, cheese and other dairy food, these fats are easily accumulated without being used efficiently due to their saturated nature. If the supply of fat is in the form of vegetable oils, except coconut and some other tropical plant fats, they are readily used in the role of energy, body construction, and other necessary metabolic functions, because of their unsaturated nature. Therefore, the intake of fat should be made in the form of vegetable oil besides natural fat contained in grains, seeds, vegetables, fruits and nuts, as well as in the form of fish and seafood, whose fat is more unsaturated in quality.

The macrobiotic way of eating which generally avoids the eating of animal food, recommending more vegetable oil than animal fat, and which recommends whole grains and vegetables as the major portion of daily food, produces a much smoother metabolism and more flexible motion of the body.

E. *The problem of vitamins*

Recent awareness of the role of vitamins encourages the belief that it is necessary to add supplemental vitamins in addition to what we are taking as daily food. However, when vitamins are added as the additional supplement to our common food, regardless of whether their origin is natural or artificial, the effect produced is chaotic rather than helpful for our body metabolism. Vitamins exist naturally in various foods and they should be consumed as a part of food together with other nutrients.

Vitamins: Yin and Yang

Yin Vitamins:

> Vitamin B_1 (antineuritic, antiberiberi vitamin—thiamine)
> Vitamin B_2 (Vitamin G, lactoflavin— riboflavin)
> Niacin (Nicotinic acid, pellagra-preventive factor, niacinamide)
> Folic Acid (Pteroylglutamic acid)
> Vitamin B_{12} (anti-pernicious anemia factor, cyanocobalamine)
> Vitamin C (antiscorbutic factor, ascorbic acid)

> Other vitamins also belong to this category, such as Pantothenic acid, Inositol, and Para-aminobenzoic acid.

Yang Vitamins:

> Vitamin A (Antixerophthalmic vitamin)
> Vitamin D (Antirachitic vitamin)
> Vitamin K (Antihemorrhagic vitamin)
> Vitamin E (Antisterility vitamin)
> Vitamin B_6 (Pyridoxine)

> Other vitamins such as Biotin and Choline also belong to this category.

Mankind has taken vitamins in that way for hundreds of thousands of years.

There are two general classes of vitamins: fat-soluble vitamins, including A, D, and K, and water-soluble vitamins, including B_1, B_2, B_{12}, C, Niacin, and Folic Acid. Fat-soluble vitamins are more yang, while water-soluble vitamins are more yin. When our general food tends to become more yin in quality, having more salad, fruits, sugars and so-called vegetarian and fruitarian practices, more volume of yang vitamins with some yin vitamins such as B_1, B_2, and B_{12} are required. If our diet becomes more yang in quality, with the consumption of meat, eggs, more salted food, and more well-cooked food, more volume of yin vitamins is required. A theory that the daily consumption of a large dose of vitamin C is necessary, through eating citrus fruits or drinking their juice, is popular among people eating much animal food; however, this is not suitable for people eating vegetarian and fruitarian diets, whose food is more yin, already rich in vitamin C.

At the same time, there is a general belief that citrus fruits are the most efficient source of vitamin C, and that vitamin B_{12} is best supplied in the form of animal food such as liver and eggs. Such belief largely depends upon commercial promotion or insufficient understanding of food composition. Many green leafy vegetables contain much more vitamin C than citrus fruits, and, contrary to popular belief, vitamin C is not destroyed so easily in cooking, unless such cooking lasts longer than 8 minutes at $100°$ Centigrade, the boiling temperature of water. Also, vitamin B_{12} is existing in many fermented food products even of vegetable quality, and in some sea vegetables. In the market, B-complex vitamins, for example, are commonly recommended for various conditions of health, but this practice has resulted from eating refined grains and other unbalanced dietary practices which do not supply vitamins naturally within each food. The macrobiotic way as practiced throughout the centuries, and which has resulted in long life among many people, nourishes us with all necessary vitamins contained in the natural form of food, in various kinds of grains, beans, land and sea vegetables, fruits, seeds, nuts, and some animal food.

F. The problem of minerals—inorganic salts

Our body contains various kinds of minerals, including calcium (Ca)—39%; phosphorous (P)—22%; potassium (K)—5%; sulphur (S)—4%; chlorine (Cl)—3%; sodium (Na)—2%; magnesium (Mg)—0.7%; iron (Fe)—0.15%; with many minute amounts of minerals such as iodine (I), manganese (Mn), copper (Cu), nickel (Ni), arsenic (As), bromine (Br), silicon (Si), selenium (Se), and others. Approximately eighty percent of our body consists of water, containing these minerals, because we have come out of the primordial ocean in the process of evolutional development, and we have taken in this mineral water resembling ancient seawater within our body in the form of the bloodstream and other body fluids.

Minerals are not only forming the bones, muscles and other structures but also, as seawater neutralizes various toxins streaming into the ocean from the land, are serving to maintain smooth metabolism by harmonizing excessive conditions of either yin or yang. For example, excessive sugar intake results in the condition of acidosis in the blood, which is neutralized by using such minerals as calcium and is discharged ultimately from our body in the form of carbon dioxide (CO_2) and water. Therefore, a constant supply of various minerals in the form of sea salt, various vegetables and other food is necessary for our daily life. Refined sea salt, pure salt, is nearly pure sodium chloride (NaCl) only, which is unsuitable for such metabolic requirements. Also, a common belief that milk and other dairy food can supply Ca more than any other food, as a reason for daily consumption of dairy food, is also unreasonable. Vegetables, especially green and white hard vegetables, contain calcium in larger volume, often more than milk products; and many sea vegetables contain many more times calcium than dairy food.

Again, these minerals should not be taken separately from our daily food but should be taken in the form of a part of our natural food.

G. *The problem of acid and alkaline*

The effect of food in relation with blood quality often raises the question of the balance between acidity and alkalinity. Our blood, under normal circumstances, should be maintained in a slightly alkaline condition, having a pH between 7.3 and 7.45. Acids are being constantly produced in the body during metabolic processes, yet the blood reaction remains relatively constant by the elimination of excessive acid conditions in the form of CO_2 through the lungs and in the form of urination by the kidneys, and through the action of buffers in the blood. In these elimination processes, especially in the buffer system, mineral compounds are being used to

---

Calcium (Ca) Content in Various Foods (per 100 grams, unit mg)
Dairy foods are known as a source of Ca, but many other foods are also rich in Ca, and often contain more than dairy foods. Following are some examples:

Dairy foods:		Seaweeds (Sea vegetables):	
Cow's milk	100–118	*Kombu* (Tangle)	800
Goat's milk	120–129	*Hijiki*	1,400
Cheese, various	94–850	*Wakame*	1,300
Vegetables:		*Arame*	1,170
Turnip greens	130	Agar-agar	400
Long radish greens	190	Seeds and Nuts:	
Mustard greens	140–183	Sesame seeds	630–1,160
Parsley	200	Sunflower seeds	120–140
Leaf—beet	100–120	Sweet almonds	234–282
Spinach	93–98	Brazil nuts	169–186
Watercress	90	Hazel nuts	186–209
Shepherd's purse	300		
Dried radish root	400		
Beans and bean products:			
Kidney beans	130		
Broad beans	100		
Soybeans	190–226		
Tofu (soybean curd)	120–128		
Fried *tofu*	300		
Congealed *tofu*	590		
Natto (fermented soybeans)	92–103		
Miso, various	70–180		

Besides those examples, many fish and seafoods are also rich in Ca.
Source: U.S. Department of Agriculture and Japan Nutritionist Association

change strong acid into weak acid. For example,

$$HCl + NaHCO_3 — NaCl + H_2CO_3$$

Hydrochloric acid (strong acid) has been replaced by carbonic acid (weak acid).

There is a belief, in relation with the problem of acid and alkaline, that food containing more acid (pH factor less than 7.3) should be avoided in daily eating, and alkaline food is more recommended. Often this belief leads people to avoid consuming whole grains because they appear more acid than alkaline before eating. In operation, the living metabolism is not so simple. Some alkaline foods such as sugar and fruits often produce an acid condition in the blood, though acid foods such as meat and eggs are also producing acid conditions. Whole cereal grains showing an acid condition in pH factor by their phosphorous compound, produce rather a weak alkaline condition in the blood and the phosphorous compound is used for buffer action to eliminate strong acids.

—Cereal grains (acid) produce alkaline
—Most vegetables (alkaline) produce alkaline
—Some vegetables, especially tropical origin (alkaline) produce acid
—Sugar (alkaline) produces acid
—Meat and other animal food (acid) produce acid
—Fat and oil (acid) produce acid
—Minerals (alkaline and acid) produce alkaline in some cases, acid in some other cases, and used for buffer in some cases

In order to understand the balance of the living mechanism of acid and alkaline, resulting from various kinds of food, it is simple and practical that we use yin and yang more than the concept of acid and alkaline: very yin and yang foods produce acid, and generally balanced quality of food produces alkaline conditions. The macrobiotic way of eating when practiced properly can secure always a slightly alkaline condition very smoothly.

Foods Containing Vitamin C (Ascorbic Acid) (Unit mg)
Citrus fruits—lemons, oranges, grapefruit, tangerine, and others—are well-known as a source of Vitamin C. Their Vitamin C contents are generally 38 to 61 mg. per edible portion 100 grams. Besides them, many vegetables are rich in Vitamin C. For example:

Broccoli	113	Kale leaves	125–186
Brussels sprout	102	Horseradish	81
Cabbage leaves	47	Mustard greens	97
Cauliflower	78	Turnip greens	139
Chives	56	Swiss chard	32
Collard leaves	92–152	Watercress	79
Cress	69		

Also, among fruits growing in the temperate region, strawberries (59) and various other berries are rich in Vitamin C.

Source: U.S. Department of Agriculture

appendix

Seven Levels of Eating

The eating manners of all the people of the world belong to one of the following seven levels, according to their levels of judgment and consciousness:

1st Level: Eating spontaneously according to appetite, without using any clear consciousness. People of this level eat whatever is available around them. Their way of living is to respond spontaneously with no thought or idea, to any external stimulus.

2nd Level: Eating according to sensory desire, including taste, smell, color and volume. People of this level are those who are following popular tastes, seeking food more satisfying to the senses. Seeking sensory pleasure and satisfaction of the desires through any venture is their way of life.

3rd Level: Eating according to emotional satisfaction. These people prefer an atmosphere and dish arrangement appealing to their sentimental comfort, often using music, candles, and certain patterns of dishes for aesthetic reasons. Some of them advocate vegetarianism for the sentimental reason that they do not wish to kill animal life.

4th Level: Eating according to intellectual justification. This way of eating is generally based upon nutritional theory including the concepts of calories, vitamins, enzymes, protein, carbohydrates, fat, minerals and many other various food components. This is the theoretical way of eating in modern society, but its defect is the lack of a large view of the biological nature of humanity in relation with the environment, and the absence of a truly comprehensive principle.

5th Level: Eating according to social conscience. This way of eating is based upon the idea of fair distribution, often with the principle of equality. At the same time, ethics and morals as well as economic consciousness controls the kinds and volume of food consumed. Socialistic control in food production and distribution belongs to this level. Also, national and international economy often administers food programs on this level.

6th Level: Eating according to ideological belief. The way of eating based upon traditional religious and spiritual teachings belongs to this level. Judaism, Hinduism, Buddhism, Taoism, Shintoism, and many other traditional teachings include dietary disciplines. This way of eating is now either blindly followed, or is ignored, in modern society.

7th Level: Eating according to free consciousness. This way is to eat according to clear intuitive judgment, exercised freely. This intuitive way of eating does not oppose any kind of food, yet automatically selects and prepares food to make the best adaptability to the environment. This way is also to eat in order to realize one's dream.

The lower levels of eating produce more disharmony between people and the natural environment, resulting in physical, mental and spiritual chaos. The higher levels of eating produce more harmonious relations with the environment. However, the ways of eating from the first to the sixth levels eventually result in disorder. Only the seventh level of eating can secure health and happiness for individuals and society as a whole. This way of eating begins from the understanding of the order of the universe and biological clarification of clouded consciousness through the practice of proper diet for some period.

chapter 4

The Way of Life for Humanity

When man becomes able to manage his food,
he expands his memory towards Infinity.
When his memory expands infinitly, his
dream develops without end. Though his
body is small, the ocean of his spirit
is boundless, beyond time and space.
It penetrates to the beginningless
beginning, and it embraces the endless end.

January, 1977

1. Practicing a Natural Way of Life

Man, as a manifestation of the infinite order of the universe, within the infinite universe, eats everything in the universe. First, according to his biological nature, as he appeared on this earth, he eats the minerals of the earth, the waters of the earth, and all biological life, as we saw in the previous chapter. Second, he eats air and the atmosphere surrounding the earth by breathing both through the respiratory system and through the entire surface of his skin. Third, he eats various sorts of vibrations, ranging from long waves to short waves, from low frequency to high frequency, through his sensory receptors and the entire surface of his body. The sense of touch deals with vibrations manifested in solid matter; the sense of taste deals with vibrations manifested in liquid form; the sense of smell deals with vibrations manifested in the form of air; the auditory sense receives vibrations transmitted through the atmosphere; and the visual sense further interprets light waves. These foods are sensory foods.

Beyond sensory food, man eats radiations and waves coming constantly from his surroundings, near and far, even from the distance of hundreds of billions of light years—including various cosmic rays. He receives them into the surface of his body and he transmutes some of them into electro-magnetic waves which he circulates through his system of meridians. They charge his trillions of cells, glands and organs, and his entire body. By this charge he moves, he digests, he breathes, he discharges and he thinks.

He eats all physicalized food—minerals, water, vegetables, animals, and air, through the front digestive and respiratory systems; and he eats the food of vibration, waves, radiation, and various rays, which are the unphysicalized and invisible environment, through the back nervous system and through the network of meridians. We may call the former physical food, and the latter spiritual food. We eat physical food only at intervals, but we eat spiritual food continuously. Physical food is taken

[75]

Fig. 29 Cosmological Chart of Food

Physical, Material Food and
Unphysicalized, Spiritual Food

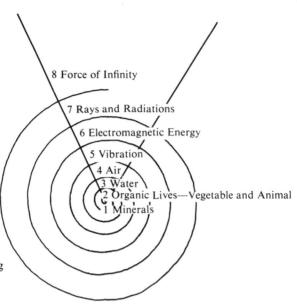

8 Force of Infinity

7 Rays and Radiations

6 Electromagnetic Energy

5 Vibration

4 Air

3 Water

2 Organic Lives—Vegetable and Animal

1 Minerals

Environments 1 through 4 are physical
and material food. Environments 5
through 8 are unphysicalized spiritual
food. The physical and material foods
are eaten through the nose and mouth,
and descend to the lungs and intestines,
while spiritual food is eaten through the
nervous systems and meridians, ascending
towards the midbrain. Both nourish the
whole body.

in limited volume, but spiritual food is taken without limit.

Between physical food and spiritual food, or material food and nonmaterial food, however, there is an antagonistic and complementary relationship in the quality and volume taken:

1. The more we eat material food, the less we eat nonmaterial food. The less we eat material food, the more we eat nonmaterial vibrational food.

2. The more we eat animal quality material food, the less we eat shorter waves in nonmaterial food, and the more we eat longer waves—the consumption of animal quality food tends to limit our perception to the immediate environment and inhibit our awareness and receptivity of the unlimited large scope of time and space.

3. The more we eat vegetable quality food, the more we receive short waves, and the less we receive longer waves—the consumption of vegetable quality food

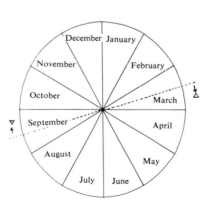

Yin and Yang of Birth Month

A person who was born between March and September in the northern hemisphere has a yang constitution because he or she spent his embryonic period mostly in the colder season, eating his mother's more yang quality of blood, which was nourished by more cooked winter food, including a larger consumption of animal food. Accordingly, a person who was born between September and March has the opposite, yin constitution. A person who has a yang constitution is generally more active in society, while a person who has a yin constitution tends to be more mental and spiritual. However, they respectively seek their opposite and are attracted to their complement, throughout their lifetime.

tends to broaden our mental and spiritual view and lessen our concern for small matters of the relative world.

Though we eat both physical and spiritual, material and nonmaterial food, we are unable to manage to directly control the quality and quantity of spiritual, nonmaterial food. However, spiritual and nonmaterial food is controlled by our regulation of the consumption of physical and material food. Therefore, how we change what we eat as our daily food determines the quality of mental, spiritual awareness we develop. We cannot directly and freely control the spiritual and nonmaterial food which comes to us, while we have complete freedom to control physical and material food: what kinds of food, how we combine various kinds, what kind of cooking is applied, how much volume is taken, how often meals are eaten. Every person among the four billion in the world exercises his freedom in what he eats and drinks. Since there are, then, four billion varieties of eating, four billion differences come out in personal conduct and behavior as well as in personal emotion and consciousness. One person is slower in his action, and another is faster in his motion; some people are more sentimental, others more intellectual; some are more conservative and others more progressive. Everyone has his own unique characteristics, everyone has his habits. All are different, and there are no two who are the same.

In order to balance our physical, mental and spiritual activities through our daily life, therefore, we have to maintain our daily food in the proper order. When we include a larger amount of animal food than we really require, our mental activities tend to become more egocentric and aggressive towards the outer world. On the other hand, if we use vegetable food almost exclusively, with a large volume of fruits, we tend to exclusivity and a defensive attitude towards any strong stimulus coming from our surroundings. A large volume of yang, such as animal food, and a large volume of yin, such as salad and fruits, hot spices, and alcohol, produce fear and exclusivity, sometimes expressed similarly, but often with an opposite expression: the more yang category of food produces a more aggressive and offensive attitude, while more yin food produces a more defensive and self-excusing tendency. The former contributes more towards a materialistic view, the latter towards the forming of spiritualism. We should balance in the middle, avoiding excessive yang and yin qualities of food; and therefore, the macrobiotic way of eating is fundamentally

---

The Secret of Noh *Plays*
(*Noh* is a more than 700-year-old religious and spiritual dance drama in Japan.)

"Furthermore he must know what the propitious times are. He must remember that a tree which bore many blossoms last year will not bear richly this year. Even in a single moment there is a time of yô (male principle) and a time of yin (female principle). No matter how hard he tries he is at the mercy of yin and yô. This is beyond his control . . .

"On the first day of a continuous three-day program should somewhat conserve his energy, because when his most important day comes he must be able to do his best in a well-written play which is one of his favorites. Even within one day's performance, when he is competing with other actors, he will naturally have a time of yin. When this happens, he should save his energy and wait for the return of a time of yô, because then his rival actors will be in a time of yin and he can take advantage of this by performing vigorously and effectively in a well-made No. If he wins in such a competition, his performance will have been the best of the day."—Excerpts from Ch. VIII, "Further Secret Instruction," in *Kadensho* (花伝書) by Ze-ami (世阿弥).

important for mental and spiritual balance.

Food results in various physical manifestations, and, at the same time, in various mental and spiritual manifestations. For this reason, it does not make sense if we expect to obtain any mental and spiritual awareness without consideration of what we are eating. Mental and spiritual teachings and their exercises are ineffective without proper practice of dietary balance. The macrobiotic way of life respects food as the essence of all surroundings, including the physical and spiritual environment, and treats it as a spiritual manifestation of the universe, as well as recognizing its physical value.

1. We should treat every tiny grain, every piece of vegetable, as a spiritual manifestation, and should never waste them in the process of choosing, preparation, cooking and eating.

2. Before and after we eat, we should dedicate our hearty gratitude for the food which has come from the infinite universe, materializing in the form of a meal, and we should dedicate our endless thanks to nature and the universe, as well as to society, which has made our existence possible at this moment. Further, we should dedicate our deep appreciation to the people who have prepared this meal, beginning from cultivation, through transportation and processing, to the final stage of the cooking and serving of the meal.

3. While we are eating, we should chew thoroughly in order to both physicalize and spiritualize what we are eating, maintaining in our mind constant self-reflection whether we are worthy to consume these foods; and maintaining our clear awareness that we shall devote our physical and spiritual activity which shall come from this food, for the benefit of society and all people, and for harmony with nature and the universe.

4. When we end our eating, we should be aware clearly that what we have shared with friends and family—eating together, drinking together—is now producing a similar quality in blood, body, thought, and movement, and we should extend this consciousness to every person living in our society, and in our world, thinking of all of them as one family of the earth and the universe.

5. During the meal, we should never leave any food remaining in the dish, and after the meal we should wash our own dishes and utensils, and keep them in beautiful order with silent thanks for their efficient service in making it possible for us to consume these foods.

From this biological nourishment which is practiced spiritually, all other aspects of living with the spirit of humbleness and modesty, and with the manner of beauty and grace, will spring up naturally.

(1) *Clothing*

When we eat macrobiotically, we begin to recover our natural sensitivity, and start to avoid synthetic unnatural clothing, especially directly touching the surface of the body. Vegetable quality materials—cotton and jute, as well as silk and other biological fabrics—become more preferred. Natural materials also secure the smoothness of our breathing metabolism, and of our heat and water metabolism through the skin. The electromagnetic charge working throughout the body is also smoothly activated with vegetable fabrics. Our taste in colors and ornaments also changes towards those which are more gentle and graceful, as we appreciate the simple beauty beyond any glamorous decoraton. Practically speaking, due to the decrease of excessive calories, fat, and liquid, garments can be kept in wearing condition for a longer period. Health and beauty become luminous through simple, natural and graceful clothing.

(2) *Dwelling*

As a result of the macrobiotic way of eating, which brings us close to nature, we begin to appreciate more wood and stone than metal and concrete for construction materials. The former tend to make the atmosphere softer and quieter, while the latter create a more hard and oppressive feeling. A peaceful mind, deep thought, and clear ideas are nourished by the more peaceful material used in our dwellings. For our furniture, desks, cabinets, closets and all other objects we use in daily life, vegetable quality materials are preferred over animal and synthetic quality materials.[1] The simpler the ornament, the better for our mind. These more natural materials used for our furniture and equipment for living are to secure our healthy life. The color of walls and curtains should also be more gentle instead of vividly distinctive. If we wish to keep our happiness—physical and spiritual—we must arrange our dwellings more in contact with nature.

(3) *Daily Contact with Nature*

Traditional ways of life in temperate climatic regions are aiming to keep our relation with nature as close as possible. The entranceways and windows of traditional homes are far larger than in modern construction, and are freely adjustable according to the change of weather. They invite more natural light into the house and rooms, and they even bring plants and soil into the rooms in the form of flower arrangements, *bon-sai, bon-kei,* and potted plants.[2] Heating in the house is kept more suitable for maintaining natural comfort and not at an unnecessarily high temperature. Even the materials used for the cooking fire are preferred to be more wood, charcoal and gas rather than petroleum, electricity, and microwave. The application of these fires is to be kept gentle and slow.

---

[1] Use of *Tatami* (畳・たたみ), *Shoji* (障子・しょうじ), and *Fusuma* (襖・ふすま): Traditional Japanese houses maintain a clear distinction between the inside and outside of the house. The house floor is elevated (more yin), constructed entirely from wood, paper and bamboo with the aid of some earth plaster (yin materials). The use of these materials brings more tranquility to one's physical and spiritual condition. Also, they use as a floor covering, *tatami* mats, made from weeds and straw. Taking off the shoes at the entrance of the house and sitting on these mats, traditionally make people's health and mind in a state of harmony with nature. *Shoji* screens and *fusuma* sliding doors, made of paper and wood, are used to divide rooms. By moving the screens or sliding the doors, room space is adjusted to maintain harmony with nature by the vegetable quality of these room dividers.

[2] *Bon-sai* and *Bon-kei: Bon-sai* (盆栽) are miniature trees and plants, planted and cared for in a pot, showing the beauty of natural life. *Bon-kei* (盆景) is natural scenery in miniature, arranged with natural plants, trees, soil, rocks, stones, and often with water. Both are cared for over many years so that people who see them can appreciate the beauty of nature to the extent that they receive a feeling of spiritual tranquility. Those *bon-sai* and *bon-kei* are one of the classical arts of the Far East, appreciated by many people for centuries.

(4) *Reasonable Use of Technological Conveniences*

Various technological applications of modern societies are giving substantial convenience to our daily life, but at the same time are hazardous to our health and spiritual well-being. An abundant use of electricity changes the atmospheric charge surrounding us, giving various effects to our physical and mental condition. Often we may notice a general fatigue, mental irritability and unnatural metabolism of body and mind produced by this unnatural atmospheric charge. Similarly, an abundant use of television, radio, and other communication instruments are giving undesirable effects to our physical and spiritual well-being. Cooking done by electricity and microwaves also gives undesirable effects to our digestion and nourishment. Synthetic materials used often in our surroundings prevent healthy relaxation. When we start to change our blood to a healthy quality by eating macrobiotically, we become naturally able to limit the use of unnatural technological comforts in our environment. This is not to deny totally the use of technology in our daily life, but rather makes us much wiser and able to sensitively choose and arrange the proper use of technological conveniences. We should avoid the use of excessive technological aids which may hinder our smooth contacts with the natural environment.

(5) *Natural Personal Care*

In addition to eating natural-organic food prepared in macrobiotic order, we should also consider the use of natural quality goods and methods in caring for our personal needs. For example, when we brush our teeth, we should avoid the use of any chemicalized and synthetic toothpaste and powder, and should use more natural materials traditionally used among many races, including sea salt, *denshi*[3], clay, and natural vegetable chlorophyll paste or powder. Similarly, when we wash and bathe our face and body, instead of using chemically colored and perfumed soap, we should use more naturally processed soap, including those of clay base or with other plant materials. In order to care for hair and skin, as well as lips and nails, we should also avoid any cosmetics and conditioners which have been processed with chemical and synthetic additives, and we should use more natural quality materials traditonally used before modern society developed. Among some traditional Asian societies, seaweed was used to care for hair; and the ancestors of European and Asian people used plant juices for coloring lips, cheeks and nails. In caring for our skin, instead of using chemically produced hand creams and skin lotions, we can use natural sesame or olive oil or natural lotions containing those oils, with excellent results. Also, for cleaning our clothing and for washing our dishes, soaps or detergents made from natural ingredients are preferred rather than artificially-made products.

Because our human nature has evolved along with the progressive change of the natural environment, we should maintain contact with nature as closely as possible.

---

[3] *Denshi* (デンシー): *Denshi* is also called "dentie." Traditionally in oriental countries, eggplant (very yin) is baked until it turns into black powder (very yang). The top end of the eggplant nearest the stem is used. This powder has been used traditionally and commonly as a tooth powder, after it is mixed with roasted unrefined sea salt (20% to 50%, depending on need). *Denshi* is excellent not only for cleaning teeth, but also for keeping gums in clean and tight condition. Because *denshi* is strongly yang, it is also used for ruptured skin or nosebleeds to contract the skin and blood capillaries, thus causing an almost immediate cessation of bleeding.

Appreciation of nature as our mother and as the source of our life is one of the most important virtues of mankind. When we respect and love our natural surroundings which create and nourish our life and growth, and we try to harmonize our existence with this natural environment, our health and spirit become the most active yet peaceful possible. The secret of longevity is within our daily life in which we are always together with nature.

2. Respect for Ancestors and Love for Offspring

Without the infinite universe and its endless order, everything and every phenomenon would not have appeared. Without the order of nature, biological life would never have come. Without ancestors, our human life would also not have existed. Everyone has parents—father and mother. Every father and mother has his and her parents. All grandparents have their parents. Our existence here and now is owing, besides to our natural environment, to our parents and ancestors which have been succeeding generation to generation beyond hundreds of thousands of years. We are at present the end manifestation of a long process of tradition—biological, psychological and spiritual—which has continued for thousands of generations.

Our respect for our parents is the beginning of all common codes of mankind. There is no one whose conduct is substantially wrong in his personal behavior and in his social relations if he respects and loves his parents. During the period we were growing up through our embryonic and childhood periods, love and care were poured upon us by our parents. Their love for their children was unconditional, and they treated their children as their own life. They were worried when their children suffered with sickness. They could not sleep during many days and weeks while the children were struggling with any physical, mental and social difficulties. When parents had their first child, and then more children, their view of life started to be formed around the development of the children. Many parents changed their dream and ambitions for the benefit of their children. Many parents worked harder than ever because of their hope that their children could be cared for well. Even when parents use harsh expressions and give hard circumstances to their children, it is seldom that they do these things because they wish to ignore their children; these are rather given to the children with the hope that the children may grow more strong from the experience of these difficult situations.

When we are growing, often we do not see the love extended to us by our parents, and when we begin to have our own children, we start to know how much love and care we have received. However, often at that time we are unable to extend our thanks to our parents because we are occupied in caring for our own children, or in various social activities; and when we reach the age when we are able to think back and understand the past care and protection of our parents, and wish to return our gratitude to them, most parents have already passed away. Parents' love and care for their children are unconditional. Therefore, children, when they grow, should respect and care for their parents unconditionally. It is a natural, universal, and common principle of human conduct. If we do not practice it, however great we are in fame, position, property, and social influence, we are worthless in the order of the universe.

Respect and care for the parents should include the following behavior:

(1)   When living with the parents, extending our daily greetings to them every morning after we get up, and every evening before retiring to sleep. When we live separately from them, we should regularly communicate with them as often as possible, informing them of what we are doing. We should try not to worry them about ourselves. We should send from time to time, monetary and material assistance, or symbols of our appreciation, however small they may be.

(2)   When parents suffer with sickness and in any difficulties, emotional, financial and social, we should extend our unconditional assistance and support. Even if we have to sacrifice our own development, comfort and prosperity, we should help unconditionally to relieve parents from any sort of suffering.

(3)   When living together with our parents, we should arrange every day if possible or as often as possible, the opportunity to be together sharing meals. At that time, we should serve the parents and should start to eat after they have started to eat. Their seats should be arranged at the most comfortable place at the head of the table. During mealtime, exchange conversation and report what you are doing, asking what can be done for the parents.

(4)   We should seek often their advice and opinions about life in general and receive their inspiration and guidance. We should also ask as much as possible to hear the experiences in life which parents had in the past years, and also the stories of ancestors —where they were living, how and what they were doing, and with what dream and spirit these ancestors were conducting their lives.

(5)   Whatever happy and joyous news we have, we should first report to the parents, before anyone else. Whatever sadness, we should try to avoid letting them know. However, the happiness and joy of the parents should be treated as our own happiness and joy; and the sadness and misery of the parents should be shared as our own sadness and misery.

In modern society, public institutions or professional homes are often used to care for aged parents, even if their children are living with healthy and prosperous conditions. It is undesirable that we arrange for our parents to stay in such institutions while we are able to be with them. Respect for our parents is not merely a monetary and material question, but a more emotional and spiritual question, and we should express it unlimitedly and unconditionally.

Through the respect of our parents, we learn about our ancestors. The spirit of our ancestors is living biologically, psychologically and spiritually within us, whether we

---

Ko-Kyo (孝経)—*The Book of Filial Piety* written by Confucius and his disciples, begins as follows: "All bodies, hair and skin have been received from Father and Mother. To keep them undamaged and unspoiled is the beginning of filial piety. Leaving our names to the future generation through our development of personality and practice of Tao (the order of the universe) is the end of filial piety." (5th century B.C.)

are aware of it or not. From our parents, we receive our biological and psychological constitution, carrying the influence of our grandparents, and, further, the influences of great-grandparents upon them. Practically seven generations are manifested within our physical, mental and spiritual constitution very clearly, and theoretically an unlimited number of generations have descended into our existence. We extend our appreciation to all ancestors through learning their histories, and if that is not possible, through making self-reflection within ourselves—since we are representing a succession of the stream of life coming down through our ancestors.

(1)   We should set a time every morning and/or every evening, if possible, to extend our prayers, to report what we are doing and to wish spiritual happiness to our ancestors, together with our dedication of endless gratitude to them. If it is not possible every morning or evening, or both, then every month or at least every year, a certain date should be specially arranged for this prayer. We may offer meals on such occasions, and such meals should not contain animal quality food. The minimum requirement of such offering should consist of grains, water, and unrefined sea salt; use the most unspoiled portion of the cooked food before serving to the family and dinner guests as the offering to the ancestral spirits, when we dedicate our prayers.[4]

(2)   We should keep any memory and any objects which our ancestors appreciated and enjoyed, as our family treasures. We should keep them with the best care and pass them on to the next generation. We should also tell our children and our grandchildren about their ancestors: their dream, their spirit, their work, and their understanding, and let them be aware of the fact that they are following these traditions.

(3)   Respect for ancestors, however, should not be limited to only several generations or even several hundred generations prior to us. Such respect should be dedicated to unlimited generations prior to our generation. Chinese people should not limit their respect for ancestors to the beginning period of China; Jewish people should not limit their respect to the time their ancestral history began; those of Scandinavian descent should not limit their respect of parents to the time of the formation of Scandinavian countries. Our respect of the traditions of the ancestors should go back far beyond the time of the beginning of written history. It should go back to the common ancestors of all people, all races, and eventually reach their common origin: nature, earth, the universe, and the life of the universe itself. Respect of ancestors ultimately becomes the same as the respect of the order of the universe,

---

[4] *Prayers for Ancestral Spirits:*   In many traditional countries among the practices of Shintoism, Buddhism, Confucianism, Taoism, and among many other religious and spiritual cultures, there are ceremonies, festivities and prayers dedicated for ancestral spirits. In traditional oriental families, in the most quiet room of the house, is usually placed the KAMI-DANA (神棚)—Shelf for spirits; the SAI-DAN (祭壇)—platform for worshipping spirits; or the BUTSU-DAN (仏壇)—miniature Buddhist temple. There they keep the names of ancestors or symbols of ancestral spirits, and daily offering of meals is made by the main members of the household. In any important event, the family and relatives gather and confer in front of this sacred place. Furthermore, on the memorial days of family members who have passed away and of important ancestors, they gather all family members, relatives and friends for special memorial ceremonies and parties either in front of the spiritual place in the house, or in the shrine or temple.

the origin of all life, and expands to the brother- and sisterhood among everyone and every being arising on this earth and appearing in this endless universe.

Love and care extended to children from parents are unconditional. Parents offer their lives totally to the development of children. Love and care of the parents are more intuitive, and similar to the instinctive nature which is common in many biological species. However, in the case of mankind, such love and care for children should not be conducted only by such biological instinct, but should be directed by more intellectual and spiritual understanding of the future of the children and their relation to human society.

(1)   Often, sentimental love and caring for children, protecting them from hardship including cold weather, material poverty, social misery and various other difficulties, tends to spoil the development of self-discipline, endurance, vitality, and understanding in children. Wise parents often arranged for their children the experience of various hardships, accompanied by the wish that they may grow into strong personalities. Sentimental parents often try to nourish their children more than is really necessary. Material wealth, high education, a comfortable household and sweet words are not necessary requirements to bring children to a wholesome adulthood. During their lifetime, children will encounter various vicissitudes with which they must develop their happiness. Therefore, wise parents first teach their children how to keep their health; second, how to judge various problems; third, how to manage by themselves the necessities of daily life; and fourth, how to behave with other people, and how to love nature and the universe. Children who have been brought up in the macrobiotic way of life have maximum adaptability without complaining. They have also maximum endurance and patience in any difficult situation without accusing others. They have also maximum courage and ambition to solve any problem, turning difficulties into new hope. On the other hand, children who have not been brought up in the macrobiotic way of life tend to resist unfamiliar circumstances, complain about an uncomfortable environment, accuse other people, and retreat from—or try to impose themselves upon—situations beyond their abilities.

(2) Parents' love and care for their children should not contain any personal expectation by which their own emotional satisfaction is rewarded. Often parents insist that their children have certain kinds of experience, learning, and occupation, based upon their own personal desire. True love and care for children is to guide the children's potentiality, whether or not it conforms to the parents' idea, through the children's own exercise of their abilities. Accordingly, parents' education for their children is to give them a biological and psychological foundation along with the understanding of their ancestors, their natures, their community and their universe. Their love and care should direct children to grow as people who are able to perform their best contribution to society according to their own dream.

(3)   Parents' education for their children is to cultivate in the depths of their children's minds a spirit of unconditional appreciation towards everyone and everything. Parents must act as models for their children by offering their own gratitude to everyone and everything in any proper occasion. For the future happiness of their children, parents must also guide them to be honest and never lie. The example

of honesty and humbleness exercised by parents in their relations with neighbors and other people automatically guides children towards the development of wholesome personalities. Parents should never be angry towards their children, and at the same time, should not show any anger against any other person in front of their children. Anger is sickness, especially if parents are angry or upset about the attitudes of their children; a faulty attitude in children indicates that the way of life, including the way of eating, that the parents have been arranging with their children, is not macrobiotically practiced. That is due to the ignorance of the parents themselves, and the children are nothing but a natural reflection of the parents' thought and conduct.

When parents and children share together the same meal properly arranged and macrobiotically prepared, their blood can maintain the same quality with health and vitality both physically and spiritually. Such parents are sharing the same thought and spirit, and they are able to understand each other without words as one family. On the other hand, parents and children who eat in different ways and in a chaotic manner, as most modern families are doing at the present time, become separated and chaotic through the influence of their blood quality upon their physical and spiritual conditions. They experience unexpectedly various physical illnesses, mental sicknesses, and emotional and intellectual conflicts, and criticize each other's view of life. The generation gap and the collapse of the family unit evolve from these different practices of eating. Children and offspring lose the spirit of their ancestors and traditions, and they become orphans isolated from love and care, and from family and nature as well.

Unless dietary traditions are practiced in a proper macrobiotic way through many

---

Emperorship in ancient China was aiming at the Tao of the King (王道). The character for King, (王), shows the top line which indicates heaven, the bottom line which indicates earth, and the line in between which indicates man and human society. The vertical line connecting them shows Tao, which is common for heaven, earth and human affairs. In other words, the meaning of the king is, that he is a person who understands and practices the order of the universe in his own life and in the larger society. The king's most important affair was to worship the order of the universe, God; and constant prayer dedicated for the happiness of people. Japan's Emperorship is still keeping that spirit. The performance of the Emperorship includes as the most important affairs, numerous ceremonies dedicated for the order of the universe and ancestral spirits, with constant prayers for people's happiness. Many such ceremonies are performed along with ceremonial practice of the macrobiotic way of eating. Because of this primary nature, Japan's Emperorship had not been disturbed by political power through her national history of over 2,000 years.

Sayings about children and the education of children, from oriental tradition:
　—Children are treasures of three worlds. (Past, present and future.)
　—If you love your child, let him travel alone.
　—The lioness kicks her child from the gulf 1,000 feet deep. (To train the baby lion in hardship.)
　—Do not shoot a mother bear accompanied by her baby.
　—A child brought up by his grandparents has a defect in his personality. (Because of extra-sweet care often given by grandparents.)
　—To know a child better, see his parents.
Also there are many such sayings in western tradition, including the well-known "spare the rod and spoil the child."

generations over hundreds of centuries, the spirit and tradition, love and dream which the ancestors have passed down to succeeding offspring continuously from the unknown ancient time to the unknown future time, shall disappear at any time, and there would be no longer a stream of blood and spirit continuing from the beginningless beginning to the endless end, even beyond the limited destiny of the human species.

The ancestors should pass down their best, with love and care dedicated to all offspring. Offspring should continue their ancestors' spirit and dream with respect and modesty, and should further develop this spirit and dream to pass on to further offspring.

3. Man and Woman

Traditionally, it is said that man represents Heaven, and woman represents Earth. This means that the male body structure is more oriented by the centripetal force which comes from the outer periphery of the atmosphere towards the center of the earth. In man, this force from heaven passes through the spiritual channel, which is running from the top of the head (center hair spiral) towards the male genital organ, the penis. In the female body structure, centrifugal force expanding from the center of the earth by the rotation of the earth is passing through from the genital organs, the vagina and uterus, upwards to the hair spiral on top of the head. Needless to say, both sexes receive both centripetal and centrifugal force—but in differing degrees. In the case of man, the predominance of heaven's force produces a taller body, smaller breasts, extended sexual organs and his psychological tendency

Fig. 30   Heaven and Earth Forces in Man and Woman

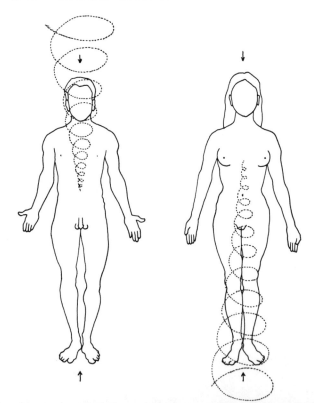

of wishing to realize his conceptual image upon the relative world of the earth. In the case of woman, the more expanding earth's force she receives through her body produces her indented sexual organs, expanded breasts, prolonged hair on the head, and her mental tendency of wishing to make order in the relative world surrounding her, towards the development of beauty and perfection.

Accordingly, the male character is more developed by taking slightly more yang food—grains, vegetables, beans, seaweed, and slightly more minerals than woman, and occasional animal food; and the female character is more benefited by taking grains, vegetables, beans, seaweed, with less salt and lighter cooking, including occasional fruits if the environment necessitates. Man manifests his character in more physical strength, conceptual intellectuality, social activity, courage and ambition, as well as the spirit that he does not mind to die for his dream. On the other hand, woman in general manifests her character more in mental understanding, emotional sensitivity, artistic gracefulness, beautifying her surroundings, gentle affection, tender care, and her spirit that she does not mind to die for love. As complemental manifestations of yin and yang of the order of the universe, man and woman share their lives together in harmony. In marriage, man and woman live together, creating harmony in the sharing of the following aspects:

(1) *Share of Food*

To develop and maintain harmony, physically, mentally and spiritually, man and woman should share the same quality of food with slight variations suitable for each sex. About seven-eighths of the food they share should be the same, and about one-eighth can be different to maintain the uniqueness of each character. For example, in macrobiotic dietary practice, the main food—grains and beans, as well as most side dishes which usually consist of vegetables and seaweed—can be the same for man and woman, but an occasional addition of a special dish may be called for: in the case of man, this may consist of fish or seafood or else more strongly-cooked vegetables; and in the case of woman, the addition of very lightly cooked leafy vegetables or fruits in small volume. Generally speaking, in temperate and warmer climates, woman can be satisfactorily nourished by all vegetable quality food, while man may have occasionally a supplement of animal food if he requires it.

Sharing such a diet, man and woman develop similar physical and mental conditions, while still maintaining their unique male and female characteristics in body and mind. Through such similarity and such differences, they can establish the most harmonious physical relationship as well as mental understanding, and they become one biologically, psychologically and spiritually.

(2) *Share of Physical Relations*

Based upon common dietary practice, physical relations become more harmonious—in attraction, in expression, and in sensory and emotional smoothness. Sexual intercourse is, very simply, to achieve the combining of heaven's centripetal force with earth's centrifugal force, passing through both connected bodies in the

---

Categorization of man and woman in ancient cosmology from which all oriental cultures have come out, identifies heaven—yang—and man; earth—yin—and woman.

form of strong waves and sparks. In such a relationship, the physical qualities of each person should be equally healthy and sensitive to the extent that their conductivities of such forces can become maximum. When we eat different food, our emotional and physical quality becomes different in its conductivity, resulting in sexual disharmony.

In physical relationships, man is generally initiating and taking the more active part, and woman is generally more receptive, elevating the feeling of oneness through her harmonizing approach. The living place may be chosen by both man and woman together, but the place of their inner relation should be prepared more comfortably by woman by her initiative, because woman is more sensitive to the surrounding conditions.

(3) *Share of Economy*

While man and woman are maintaining separate arrangements in their monetary and material affairs, their marriage is not yet accomplished. Home economy, except for business and public affairs, should be kept either by both or by one party, with unconditional trust. Larger events related to social activities may be managed by either party who is more connected to such social affairs, but most of the home economy should be managed by woman, who is usually at the center of the household. The wise husband gives all of his personal income to his trusted wife, and she manages it, including giving her husband a daily allowance for his necessities. Man should develop full trust in woman's management of home economy, and woman, responding to such trust, should manage carefully the household expenditures. Man should be generous and embracing in his attitude toward circumstances arising in his relation with woman, and woman should be modest and sympathetic in her relation with man.

(4) *Share of Families, Relatives, and Friends*

At the time of entering into the marriage relation, man and woman should consider the partner's parents as his or her own parents, the partner's brothers and sisters as his or her own brothers and sisters, and the partner's relatives as his or her own. In the exact same manner that one extends love and respect to his or her own families, one should extend love and respect to the partner's family.

   a. Learn the family history and background, and have a good understanding of the traditions of the partner's family.

Socrates says: "Anyway, marry. If your wife is good, you will be happy. If your wife is not good, you will become a philosopher." (5th Century B.C.)
Michio Kushi adds: "Anyway, marry. If your husband is good, you are happy. If your husband is not good, you will become a saint."

"Man and woman do not sit together after the age of seven."—Discourse of Confucius. (5th century B.C.)
That is, man and woman are developing their different physical and mental constitutions more distinctively after the age of seven. Accordingly, their education should begin to differ, especially in the learning of their respective life activities: man for more active social expression, woman for more gentle and artistic expression. Though many parts of their education still continue in the same manner, separation until the mating age has been considered very helpful to develop their respective unique characters which later become supportive of each other throughout their lives.

b. Learn from the partner's parents about the babyhood and childhood of the partner and have an understanding of the partner's character, personality, habits, and way of thinking.

c. Keep close relations through frequent visits or correspondence with the partner's family, and have an understanding of what is going on among them, being ready to extend any assistance necessary for them, and making active participation in the partner's family occasions.

d. Any sad events in the partner's family should be fully sympathized and attended to wholeheartedly, sharing in the family's sadness. In happy occasions in the partner's family, their joy should be shared from the heart, and congratulations should be extended to the partner's family.

e. Any important occasion such as pregnancy, delivery, sickness, success and failure in social activities, and others, should be reported to the partner's family—conflicts in married life which may arise between man and woman not excepted. One's own parents or family should not only be consulted—but also the partner's family and relatives.

Similarly, all friends of the partner should be considered as one's own friends, and as the partner treats them, he or she should also treat them. In any gathering with those friends which the partner may join, he or she should also participate. The friendship and understanding of each of such friends should be thoroughly developed. The partner's seniors should be respected as if they are his or her own seniors, and the partner's juniors should be loved and cared for as if his or her own juniors.

(5) *Share of Dream*

Everyone has a direction in his or her life. Every married man and woman should have the same dreams to be shared together. The way to approach and the way to carry out such dream may differ due to the complemental nature of man and woman. Such approach and methods to carry out should be supporting each other in the achievement of the dream: man, from his way, and woman from her way. Man and woman, however, should continuously develop their dream beyond the limited level of sensory and sentimental satisfaction. Such sensory and sentimental dreams as having a sweet home only for themselves, offering the best opportunities for their children, accumulating material wealth, seeking social power—are limited as dreams which man and woman may pursue together throughout their whole life. When those dreams are reached to a certain extent, the meaning of togetherness is lost, and there co-operative living reaches a dead end. Through their own experiences,

---

"The Teaching of the Three Followings"—"Woman should follow her father during her youth; she should follow her husband after she marries; she should follow her children when she becomes old."—Ekiken Kaibara—"The Teaching to Women and Children." (17th century.) This traditional saying is not intending to put woman into a state of slavery to man; its true intention is that woman has such an important role to create the health and happiness of everyone, that she should not be disturbed by various conflicting events arising in society.

Simon Peter said to them: "Let Mary go out from among us because women are not worthy of the Life." (In the *Gospel According to Thomas*; Log. 114.)
Michio Kushi says: "Let woman sit in the center among us because she is creating Life."

through their own learning, through their constant seeking, man and woman should continuously evolve their dream from the limited sensory-sentimental satisfaction to intellectual, philosophical fulfillment, and further, towards the endless dream for many people and the larger society. As they develop such a dream, their relationship would never become tired, mentally and spiritually, and their marriage would continue until the end of their lives. When they began to live together, they might have worked only for sensory and emotional satisfaction, but when man and woman live together, they have endless possibility toward future development, as they represent heaven and earth. By developing their dream, the meaning of their togetherness evolves naturally toward endless spiritual nature.

Woman is biologically superior to man. Her superiority is demonstrated very evidently in the following points:

1. With less animal quality food and more vegetable quality food, woman can maintain her health; this shows her ability of biological transmutation.
2. Women are able to live longer than men, three to four years on the average in most parts of the world, which shows woman's adaptability to the environment as superior to man's.
3. Woman usually requires less volume and variety of foods, demonstrating her more effective utilization of foods.
4. Woman has less body hair than man. In the biological world, more body hair indicates less biological development, as a general principle.[5]
5. Women are able to transmute their food into their body and reproductive cells, the ova, out of which they further are able to develop babies in their uterus, while men are unable to change their food into babies beyond the stage of their reproductive cells, the sperm.

These unique characteristics, in addition to many others, demonstrate woman's biological superiority to man. Accordingly, due to her more progressed development, woman has been traditionally a master of the biological care of humanity. The creation of life, not only their own babies but for their families and children, has been practiced through their preparation of daily food. Because of her judgment, she is able to prepare daily, dishes combining various factors of nourishment from nature, and offer them to her partners, children, and friends as harmonious food which would produce their health, energy, thought and activity, mind and spirituality, and moreover, culture and civilization.

In the event woman would not practice her central role in the creation of biological destiny, family and society, the country and the world would inevitably

---

[5] *Ke-Mono* (毛物). In oriental countries, especially the Far East, the word *Ke-Mono* (hairy animal —KE meaning "hair," and MONO meaning "living being") means "beast of wild character," and this expression is often used to indicate a lower grade of species.

"It is difficult to educate women and people with small minds."—Discourse of Confucius (5th century B.C.)

Traditionally, this was interpreted to mean that woman is unable to learn and comprehend. However, the real meaning of this saying is that woman is natively intuitive and understands many aspects of life, while man needs more learning through experience and studies. Therefore, when man tries to "educate" woman, it is often difficult to make her understand his point of view.

decline: many families would decompose. Children would scatter, and societies would be full of sickness, physical and mental. The world would fall into chaos and misery, and even the entire human race would move toward extinction. Wherever woman continues to prepare food macrobiotically, families and people would become healthier and healthier in body and spirit, and society would continue to develop and prosper. Wherever woman gives up the macrobiotic preparation of food, people would start to suffer from various miseries, and society would decline.

On the other hand, man is generally more idealistic, using his intellectual, conceptual thinking and organizing ability, as well as his physical vitality and spirit of adventure. In some sense, man is much more of a dreamer than woman, who is more practical in many ways. Men are often very curious, inventive and ambitious. Man begins with his idea and dream, and ends by realizing it in society. Without the spirit of adventure of man, society and the world would not develop. Men are the promoters and actors on stage to perform various roles in the theater of human drama. Men choose their roles with free choice, and act with their image, decorating the human world with interesting vicissitudes. Peace and war, rise and fall, construction and destruction, progress and retreat, challenge and response, and many other affairs in the human drama are played largely by man.

However great a man's action is, or however small his role is, all actors in this theater upon the earth are produced and directed by their mothers, wives, and mistresses who would prepare their biological, psychological qualities through their daily preparation of meals, as well as through their offering of love and care.

Therefore, man should prepare for woman the most suitable environment where she can perform her unique ability as a center of biological development, without limitation, and man should completely surrender to whatever she prepares for him.

And woman should design with her image and prepare with her grace, the most harmonious meal along with love and care for man; and through this, men would continue to develop their dreams unlimitedly, and would continue to realize them upon the earth.

4. Society and Nature

When we eat a part of our environment, transforming it into our body, mind, and spirit, we start to construct society with other people through our image. Society is a reflection of what we think and what we eat. Society is our production, and nature is our origin. Therefore, we maintain our society as the most wonderful art which we can share with other people, and we respect nature as the parent of every person.

Your Sweetheart Is Killing You
Your sweetheart calls you "honey" and never calls you "brown rice" or "whole wheat bread." This is the beginning of murdering you. You are served beautifully decorated, delicious dishes which are loaded with sugar, cream, and spices. And when you become sick by eating them, you are served out-of-season fruits, chemicalized chocolates, and sweetened candies for consolation. When you are killed because of them, your left-over money is spent by your "honey" for another sweet purpose. Our life is so wonderfully interesting, full of adventures!—Michio Kushi

People who have come out through millions of billions of years from the infinite universe, appearing as members of our society at this time and in this place, are all brothers and sisters who share the same origin—Infinity—and who share the same parents—the natural environment. We share also our future destinies with these brothers and sisters, for we all return to nature and the infinite universe—our parents and our origin.

Therefore, unconditional respect and love among people are our natural instinct and intuitive common sense if we are following the natural order through flexible adaptation to the changing environment by the proper preparation of what we consume as our food. Especially when we eat similar foods which are traditionally practiced and universally practiced throughout different regions according to macrobiotic principles, every person in our society would share the similar quality of blood and health, mind and thought, spirit and dream. We are able to understand each other without difficulty, and we are able to communicate whatever we think without hesitation. Such society is in a real sense a free society, and the natural order of harmony and peace among people would be maintained automatically.

In such a society, elders are naturally maintaining their social status similar to that of grandparents, parents, uncles and aunts. All elders should extend their love and care to all younger people without discrimination. They should consider all children of the community as their own children, all youngers as their own younger brothers and sisters. They should extend their encouragement to the younger generation to develop their dreams towards realization. They should extend consolation to the younger generation when they are in despair and in need. They should give inspiration to the younger generation towards the understanding of life and the development of happiness. They should offer assistance to the younger generation when it is needed for their progress. They should be guides for the younger generation in the pursuit of their freedom. The elders should especially watch over the health of the younger generation and lead them towards the development of an endless dream.

On the other hand, the younger generation, even of only one year difference, should respect their elders, listening to their advice, learning from their experiences, receiving their inspiration, understanding their background, and trying to continue to realize their ongoing dream. When the elders become very old, as they cared for their juniors, the younger generation should care for the elders as if they were their

---

The Council of Elders: In ancient society more than 2,000 years ago, there were Councils of Elders among many different people including the Celts, Jewish people, Chinese, Japanese, Indians and American Indians. Elders were considered wiser than the juniors through their experience, and any conflict among people was submitted to the Council of Elders for arbitration. Often in such occasions, elders gave advice on the principles of the way of life, and practical suggestions on how to solve the problem. Such councils also acted, often, as a government to set general policy for communities. Those elders were also the teachers of the way of life to every member of the community. They were not elected by people but were more naturally selected according to their experiences and understanding developed through years of life.

"Real man sorrows prior to everyone else, and rejoices after everyone else."—ancient saying in China.

own parents; not only with spiritual support and material assistance, but also, the maintenance of health and prolongation of life should be wished for the elders and facilitated by the younger people as much as possible.

Our human relations in both private and public affairs should be based upon mutual understanding. Public education based upon love and respect for all neighbors is essential for our growing period. Again, such understanding should not be taught conceptually, but should be nourished naturally through the biological and biochemical improvement of our quality of consciousness through consuming better quality food. Principles for human relations with neighboring people as well as with people who are living at a distance, include:

1. Consciousness of brother- and sisterhood among all people.
2. The respect, love and care essential for mutual living.
3. No complaints and no accusations regarding whatever is happening among ourselves and others.
4. Spirit of gratitude for whatever we receive, material and spiritual, and spirit of apology for whatever we may do which affects other people's lives, through our thought and conduct.

If there is one person in a community who understands the order of the universe and practices the macrobiotic way of life, his community will become better. If there is no such person, the community would eventually become chaotic, with people complaining to others, accusing each other, defending themselves against any other person and event. If we use others for the purpose of personal profit-making, especially in the material world, we would be used by others for the same purpose. If we put the happiness of others before our own happiness, others would put our happiness before their own happiness.

However, our harmonious relations with all other people are depending upon how we are practicing the way of life according to the order of the universe. In other words, unless we keep our physical and mental conditions in accord with the natural cycles of the environment, we do not enjoy peaceful relations with others. Therefore, we should feel, beyond anything else, that nature and the universe are our parents. Our adaptation to the changing natural environment is the root of our respect of traditions and elders, our love for other people and for our juniors, and our care of everyone and everything, including our own daily life.

1. Let us keep a spirit of endless marvel at the immeasurable beauty and perpetual order of nature and the universe, and let us keep a constant sense of marvel about how we have come from the infinite universe, physicalizing ourselves upon this earth at this time as members of the human race.
2. Let us keep a spirit of endless appreciation for nature and the universe, including all natural phenomena and for the numerous lives which have lived, are presently living, and shall be living, with us. Let us keep our gratitude for mountains and rivers, land and ocean, trees and flowers, birds and fishes, animals and vegetables, the sky and the stars.
3. When we come close to misery of any sort, let us remember that nature and the universe are still constantly cycling, and our miseries are caused by nothing more than our lack of harmony with them.

4. Let us admire the wonders of nature and the universe, including all inhabitants within them, and devote our prayers and joy in them through occasional events, festivities and ceremonies as well as self-reflection to be made deeply within our mind.

5. Let us keep nature surrounding us, the forests and soil, hills and rivers, air and lakes, ocean and land, as plentiful as they have been, as prosperous as they have been, as beautiful as they have been. When we use a part of them, we should devote our prayers and appreciation to them, and use them modestly; and we should restore such used portions to their original condition.

In many traditional cultures throughout the world, there were a variety of festivals and ceremonies dedicated to nature or the spirit of nature. Many ancient calendars set the days for these events, such as the day for the sun, the day for the moon, the day for the stars, and others.[6] They also symbolized in the image of gods and spirits, various phenomena of nature as we see in ancient mythologies in such places as Sumer, Greece, Rome, India, Japan, China, Scandinavia, the Celtic culture, and the ancient inhabitants in North and South America. Such appreciation for nature and natural phenomena is one of the most universal and commonly existing attitudes in the depths of our tradition, as our ancestors were practicing their daily life together with the natural cycles of change.

In the modern age, especially since scientific analytical observation began around the 16th century, such native intuition extending appreciation to the natural environment has declined rapidly. The desire to use the natural environment for purely human benefit or profit-making purposes has overruled that traditional spirit of harmonizing ourselves with nature. Such modern mentality has resulted in the destruction of nature—our parent—producing chemicalized soil, contaminated water, and a polluted atmosphere. Large-scale industrial production has brought material prosperity to our society through the spoiling of our natural resources and the impoverishing of our environment. This, in turn, is destroying the foundation of our biological life, and the very existence of humanity itself. The macrobiotic way of life suggests that we need to deeply self-reflect regarding our own modern thought and conduct, as well as regarding the whole orientation of the entire modern civilization, for the health, happiness, and endless existence of mankind on this earth and within this universe.

---

[6] *Events for the Appreciation of Nature:* Such modern customs in America as May Day, Arbor Day, Thanksgiving Day and many regional festivals, should be kept as traditions with the addition of a spirit of appreciation of nature. In many European countries there are such traditional days of natural celebration and appreciation. In Japan, such days include the Day for Prayer for the Sun (Jan. 1), Peach Flower Day (March 3), the Cherry Blossom Festival (late March to April), Peony Day (May 5), Star Night Festival (July 7), Lunar Festival (Sept. 9), and the Chrysanthemum Festival (Nov. 11), as well as spring and autumn thanksgiving ceremonies dedicated for rice and other foods on the days of the eqinoxes.

5. The Spirit of Macrobiotics

When we understand our origin and our future—how we have come from One Infinity to this relative world through physicalization according to the order of the universe, and how we are starting to return to Infinity again after we live as one of the human beings on this earth, and we marvel at this infinite order of life in its process and mechanism, its perpetual movement continuing from the beginningless beginning to the endless end—we start to wonder why we have come to this earth and for what purpose. Our dream of what we wish to do depends upon our memory of how we have come and from where. Without memory there is no dream; without dream there is no life. Because we have always our unidentifiable, undifferentiated, and undetermined infinite ocean of memory, we are able to image, dream, will, judge, and think.

Our life on this small planet earth is one infinitesimal process in the endless stream of the infinite life of the universe, a geometrical point in the boundless space of the infinite ocean of the universe. This life, therefore, arises, changes, moves, declines, and disappears within this universe according to its perpetual order. Our life in this space and time is a faint wave which is governed by the order of the universe, yin and yang.

The principles of our macrobiotic way of life are simply the human interpretation of the order of the universe.

(1) *Have Unconditional Faith in the Order of the Universe*

In our daily life, our sensory, emotional, intellectual and social consciousness often guide us into an illusional view of the world. We tend to think we are able to live forever, that our society would continue to develop forever, our love and friendships last forever. We also tend to think that something is right, something else is wrong, this is good, that is bad, this is beautiful, that is ugly, this is difficult, that is easy. However, all of these relative judgments are due to our limited consciousness which is unable to see endless change, from the beginningless beginning to the endless end. Relative value, whether expressed in money, matter, praise, position, fame, or glory, shall fade away very soon. What we are able to do beyond these vicissitudes of ephemerality is to have infinite faith in the order of the universe, which is eternally unchanging. We should not let our emotions and our senses rule the destiny of our life; let us lead our life by our natural intuition harmoniously working with the order of the universe.

(2) *Non-Credo*

This relative world, especially human society, is full of fallacies. We tend to believe, without experience and understanding, whatever is conceived and interpreted by our relative senses. Education, promotion, and advertisement are teaching us constantly to believe what we really do not know ourselves. Science and religion are also worlds of belief in what we really do not know. The concept of social systems, organization and administration planned artificially, is also the world of belief in what we really do not know. Do not imitate theories and assumptions which others have developed. Do not enslave your freedom with illusions and mysteries. Let us enjoy a spirit of non-credo, and let us seek endlessly through our own experience and understanding what is clear and what is not clear, what is real and what is unreal.

(3) Be Our Own Master

When we have come to this world as human beings, we must exercise our own judgment in whatever we do in this world. We have chosen this place and this time by ourselves, and we are totally responsible ourselves for anything we are doing as a mature person. When we are sick, it is caused by our ignorance of how to behave according to the laws of nature—eating the wrong food, having the wrong conduct, behaving in a wrong manner. When we are in misery, it is caused by our wrong judgment, which may come from a way of life out of harmony with the environment. Sickness, accident, miseries and any other difficulties can be turned into health, well-being and happiness through only the change of our own thought and conduct. No one else can change them in our behalf—we must initiate changes ourselves. We may receive advice, suggestions and guidance, but it is we who should act as the master of our own destiny.

(4) We Are Ignorant

When we reflect upon ourselves, what we are thinking, what we are doing in our daily life, we know our ignorance. Ignorance of life, ignorance of ourselves, ignorance of others, ignorance of nature, and ignorance of everything. Most of us do not even know what is happening to us tomorrow, how our destiny is changing in one year, and when our death is coming to us. We do not know how to keep our health, how to be joyous and how to become happy. We do not even know what we should eat, how we should breathe, what we should think, and how we should speak. We do not know whether what we think real, is true, and whether what we think good, is truly good. It is an endless dilemma and continuous disappointment when

---

"This world is full of lies and fallacies, and there is no truth." SHINRAN (親鸞) (13th century): "*The Book of Marvels*" (TAN-NI-SHO) (歎異抄)

Question: Is it worthwhile to follow masters, gurus, and teachers?
Answer: It is worthwhile to listen to them, but it is not worthwhile to follow them unless you master yourself, because no one else can eat for you, chew for you, breathe for you, think for you, act for you, or even sit on the toilet for you, other than yourself.

Question: The coming of the Messiah has been predicted by many prophets for a long period. When the Messiah comes, is our salvation achieved from this misery?
Answer: The Messiah never comes under the name of "Messiah." The Messiah is not a person who comes to some place at some time. When you talk about salvation, you are forgetting this infinite universe and its endless order, within which you are born and which is always in front of you. The awareness that you are a manifestation of this infinite universe is the true Messiah, and when you know yourself, you save yourself, finding that you are within the endless happiness of life.

The Spirit of Nothingness (Mu, 無):   Nothingness is the central concept in the spiritual training of Zen and other oriental philosophies. The state of nothingness is that we adapt freely to constantly changing circumstances by recognizing that we are ignorant, and whatever we do becomes in vain. The total surrender of ego is equal to total acceptance of surroundings which is extending to the order of the universe. To live with the spirit of nothingness is to live in the way of life according to the order of the universe.

we know what we wish to achieve, and produce the opposite result. We do not know why we came to this world, or what we should do in our life. We are always ignorant, and the more we learn, the more we become ignorant. To know that we are ignorant is the beginning of our awareness of what life is, and the beginning of our understanding of what we are. Our way of life which guides us towards true happiness comes from our deep reflection that we are ignorant. Because we are ignorant, we have to surrender unconditionally to the order of the universe. Because we are ignorant, we have to accept whatever happens around us as our responsibility. Because we are ignorant, we have to adapt to our surroundings and environment. Being humble and modest by making ourselves the last, even to the extent that we are nothing, is the shortest way to have complete freedom of life.

(5) *We Are What We Eat*

When we know that we are ignorant and submit ourselves to the hand of nature and the order of the universe, we start to understand that whatever we are taking in the form of food as well as any other environmental factors—water, air, vibrations, radiations and cosmic rays—is changing us. We are what we eat. We are a phantom of what we take in. We are a transformation of our environment, a manifestation of this universe. We eat, therefore we exist. We eat, therefore we think; we eat, therefore we move; and we eat, therefore we live. Our systems, organs, tissues, cells, molecules and atoms within our body have all come from our external world. Without food, that is, without our environment, all of our living phenomena would not continue. By changing what we take in, we change ourselves—body, mind, and spirit, and even society, culture and civilization. When we have difficulties, we should seek the cause in what we eat. When we have happiness, we understand that its origin is in our food. Those who know this become masters of their life destinies. Those who know this are free men, and those who do not know this are in slavery.

(6) *Be Grateful for Difficulties*

This world and this life are proceeding and changing paradoxically. We seek comfort; comfort produces ease; ease produces weakness; weakness produces poverty, and poverty produces difficulty. Our seeking of comfort ends by producing difficulty. When we end with difficulty, we start to seek comfort again. Therefore, comfort weakens us, and difficulties strengthen us. Poverty and cold, sickness and misery, hunger and war are all strengthening us physically, mentally and spiritually. Whenever there is no difficulty, there is no development. If we avoid such difficulties, we eventually become weaker and decline after momentary comfort. Let us welcome at any time, any sort of difficulties. Let us appreciate them as our teachers.

When we climb a mountain, the more we experience hardship, the greater joy we have when we reach the top. When we are involved in war, the more miseries we

---

Question: Does the macrobiotic way of life intend to deny such modern industrial food as sugar, soft drinks, chemical additives and monosodium glutamate?

Answer: No. The macrobiotic way of life greatly appreciates such industries, as they may produce harmful effects for our health, and because of their development we are able to more clearly understand how we should maintain our health and deepen our appreciation for the true way of life for everyone's happiness.

experience around us, the larger appreciation we would have when peace comes. When we suffer with sickness, the more serious the sickness is, the greater spirit of appreciation we would have when we restore our health. Difficulties are truly the cause of our happiness, and avoiding them is really the cause of our unhappiness. In order to be happy continuously, we should continue to put ourselves in endless difficulties.

(7) *Our Enemy Is Our Friend*

In this world there is a great variety of people; they are all our brothers and sisters sharing the same dream, the same future, and the same earth. Among them we like some people, and we do not like some others. We love some people, and we hate others. Some are our friends, and some are our enemies. When we are with those whom we prefer as our friends, we are in comfort and pleasure, and when we are with those who are our enemies, we are in tension and hardship. We consider people who give us sweet words of consolation and loving supportive care, to be our friends; but if we live only with them we become weaker, like a plant in a greenhouse. When the snows and the storms come, we wither and die. On the other hand, the enemy who accuses and attacks us, makes us cautious in action, deliberate in thought, and stronger in our abilities. We develop our strength in body and mind because of the existence of our enemy. We should be grateful to our enemies. We should be thankful for their antagonism; because they are antagonistic, they are complementary to us. They see what we cannot see. They have what we do not have. They know what we do not know. Therefore, make your enemy as your best friend. If we change our enemy into our friend, we can realize our happiness as well as our enemy's happiness.

(8) *The Last Becomes the First; The First Becomes the Last*

The endless movement of the universe, including our relative world, brings constant change from one state to another, and a return always to the previous state. Yin changes into yang, yang changes into yin. Yin produces yang, yang produces yin. The cycle of each day brings a repeating alternation of light and darkness; and of each year, an alternation of warm seasons and cold seasons. Cycles in celestial change include the cycles of solar activity, the cycle of the wobbling motion of the earth, the cycle of the motion of the solar system within the Milky Way Galaxy.

Question: Which is right, capitalism or communism?

Answer: Neither is right nor wrong. They are antagonistic, therefore, complementary. Because of the development of capitalism, communism has developed its meaning. Because of communism, capitalism is more appreciated by the people who support it. They should not destroy one another. They should develop as friends supporting each other as two different manifestations of human economical activity.

The Way of CHU-YO (中庸): CHU (中)="middle," and YO (庸)="deliberate consideration." The way of CHU-YO is to keep the middle road, balancing yin and yang, avoiding both extremes. For example, when we manage our affairs, we try to avoid rapid expansion as well as rapid contraction, and we try to avoid rapid change, taking instead a more gradual course. Keeping the middle road, avoiding extreme success and failure, and staying in a more common and ordinary state, is the Tao to manage our life. This has been a common understanding among the people of the Orient, and we can see many similar ideas and traditions among the cultures of the West.

A society begins; then, it ends; then it begins again and ends again. Life begins with birth and ends at death; but from death, new life begins. Every phenomenon expanding outward, eventually contracts towards the center, and when it contracts, it begins to expand again. Therefore, the beginning is the end, and the end is the beginning: the first is the last, and the last is the first. Alpha is omega, omega is alpha.

When we are at the foot of the mountain, we are able to reach the top. When we are at the bottom of society, we will eventually attain the top of society. When we reach the top of society, we must inevitably decline towards the bottom. The rich become the poor, the poor become the rich; the wise become the foolish, the foolish become the wise. Sickness produces health, and health produces sickness. War changes into peace; peace changes into war. The taller the tree is, the stronger is the wind which blows through its high branches. The lower the grass is, the gentler the breeze which touches it. Therefore, if we stay behind people, we never receive any strong attack or opposition, and if we stay at a low level we never experience falling down. Therefore, if we become higher, we should bow to more people, and at that time, continuing to live in the spirit of modesty and humbleness, we harmonize our destiny: the last becomes first, the first becomes last. When we become lower, we should keep our ambitious and adventurous spirit, which is making harmony in our life among the vicissitudes of this relative world.

(9)   *One Grain, Ten Thousand Grains*

Nature and the universe produce constantly within themselves two out of one, three or four out of two, and many out of three or four. Perpetual differentiation as well as perpetual gathering is the order of the universe. This universe in which we live is expanding constantly, as we know through our modern knowledge. One seed produces hundreds of seeds; hundreds of seeds produce thousands of seeds; thousands of seeds produce millions of seeds. One grain—ten thousands grains is the natural order and work of life.

When we receive one piece of bread or one bowl of rice, we ourselves produce thousands of pieces of bread, thousands of bowls of rice, and return them to the persons who offered us a piece of bread or a bowl of rice—and to many thousands of other people as well. When we learn any useful thing, we distribute it to thousands of people. Give, give, and endlessly give is the most important principle of life in order to make ourselves happy, and to make thousands of people live in happiness. When we eat, we must distribute whatever we take in. If we do not do this, we cannot eat any further. Life is receiving and giving; and the more we give, the more we

---

Day for One Grain—Ten Thousand Grains: In the traditional calendar which has been used in China, Korea and Japan since unknown thousands of years ago, two or three days in each month have always been arranged to celebrate the spirit of One Grain, Ten Thousand Grains. On those days, people are encouraged to be grateful for what they have received, to whomever has cared for them, and to return their gratitude to them, as well as to try to help others.

The story of Jesus breaking and distributing a few loaves of bread for a crowd of thousands of people (Matt. 14: 14–21), is a symbolic teaching of the spirit of One Grain, Ten Thousand Grains.

receive. When we keep ourselves busy from morning to evening, day and night, with the practice of the spirit of one grain—ten thousand grains, we are living together with the expanding universe, and this is the essential way for our endless happiness.

appendix

Overpopulation and Food

The increase in world population was gradual and fairly constant until the late 19th century, but since that time, population has begun to increase logarithmically, particularly in modern societies. For this reason, from the time of Malthus's population theory, there has developed a widespread belief that food would become too scarce to meet the rapidly increasing population. Various programs have been adopted by many national governments, including the recommendation of birth control and legalized abortion. However, the assumption that the increase of population would cause a scarcity of food is the inverse of what would actually happen. Population increases because of increasing production of food; and when food becomes less available, the population would naturally decrease.

The explosive increase of population from the late 19th century up to the present has been caused by the more active international trading of food between different continents and climatic regions. At the same time, the increase of population, which is a manifestation of a yin tendency, has been accelerated by the wider use of yin food in modern society. Such foods include, notably, refined grains, sugar, and sugar-treated food, semi-treated food, semi-tropical and tropical fruits, dairy food, potatoes, tomatoes, and chemically treated foods. If dietary practice is returned to more traditional ways, depending mainly upon regional products, according to climate and geographical region, the population would eventually become stable, as we experienced for thousands of years in the past.

Remarks on Birth Control

(1) *The Birth Control Pill:*   While progesterone is more yang, estrogen, a principal female hormone, is yin. Excessive doses of estrogen hinder the formation of eggs, which are made by the yang, inward motion of follicles in the ovaries. However, repeated overdoses of estrogen also give various yin effects throughout the woman's body, because it is carried by the circulation of blood and body fluids. These effects include headaches due to expansion of the brain cells; loss of mental clarity, caused by gradual expansion of the inner midbrain region; irregular heart palpitation, caused by gradual expansion of heart and blood vessels; gradual weakening of the functions of yang organs such as the liver, kidneys, and spleen; gradual irritation of the parasympathetic nerve function; and other similar effects. These yin conditions may manifest differently from person to person, because of differences in constitution, dietary practice, and living conditions. Some women do not feel these effects, while others experience them more noticeably. It is not recommended for any woman to take this birth control measure.

(2) *Intra-Uterine Device (I.U.D.):*   In this method, artificial obstacles of various shapes, made of either metallic or synthetic materials, are inserted within the uterus. Within the uterus, there is a constant electromagnetic flow which is generated around the so-called

hara region, the inner depths of the uterus. This electromagnetic flow charging the fertilized egg keeps the embryo alive and growing. The inserted obstacles disturb the normal pattern of this electromagnetic flow, resulting in the hindering of embryonic growth. Moreover, this method also disturbs the electromagnetic current flowing through the entire body, including KI flow through the meridians. As a result, the functions of various organs governed by electromagnetic energy flow, are directly and indirectly disturbed. This tends to cause general fatigue and emotional irritability for no other particular reason. Also, the natural mechanical response of the body is to eliminate unnatural obstacles from the uterus, and this impulse indirectly causes physical and emotional tension and disharmony, as long as the I.U.D. remains in the uterus. In order to maintain a peaceful and harmonious physical and emotional balance, it is not recommended to use the I.U.D.

(3) *Diaphragm with Foam or Jelly:* The use of a diaphragm is much safer than the above two methods of birth control, for physical and mental health. However, the use of foam or jelly which are chemically synthesized and extremely yin, causes undesirable effects, being absorbed through the wall of the vagina and uterus into the body fluid and bloodstreams. Although such effects are minor, frequently repeated use would create allergic conditions, and eventually nervousness and fatigue. It is advisable to douche with warm salty water after the use of a diaphragm with foam or jelly.

(4) *Condom:* A condom is used by the man to prevent ejaculated sperm from streaming into the vagina and uterus. This method is much safer for the health, especially in the case of woman. However, the defect of this method is that it allows no complete physical-emotional satisfaction in sexual intercourse for either party, preventing the stimulation given to the sensitive inner walls of the vagina and uterus by the ejaculated stream of sperm and sexual fluids from the man.

(5) *Natural Birth Control:* The method of birth control which is safest for mental and physical health is birth control according to the natural cycle of the ovulation period. A few days before and after the time of ovulation, usual intercourse should be avoided since the fertilizing ability of the sperm is generally two days, though they may survive as long as 14 days. In order to practice this method, however, one needs to know the exact time of ovulation, and this is only possible when the menstrual cycle is regular. Macrobiotic dietary practice and healthy overall way of life recovers the menstrual cycle from irregularity to an exact 28-day cycle following the motion of the moon. Therefore, it is possible to have natural birth control within a macrobiotic way of life.

(6) *Other Artificial Birth Control:* Because of harmful side effects produced by birth control pills, I.U.D.s, and other methods, researchers are trying to find a better solution. However, any other artificial method than natural birth control would give some degree of side effects, for shorter or longer periods. Immunization, vasectomy, and a once-a-month pill or periodical injections—all of these methods as well as any possible methods developed in the future would all give side effects, simply because they would be unnatural and foreign to the human metabolism.

In a large sense, from the view of the order of the universe, worrying about pregnancy is mental sickness, called schizophrenia. Conception is in the natural order as well as birth and death. Fear of conception and overpopulation can exist only as a delusion, among those people who are not living according to the order of nature, and who are following dietary practices out of harmony with the environment.

Proper and Improper Use of Food

If we know the order of nature and the natural characteristics of various foods—both animal and vegetable foods, their yin and yang qualities—we are able to use all foods as well as all plants and animals surrounding us for their proper medicinal uses. Food itself is medicine, but at the same time, the particular qualities of certain foods can serve as special medicines for certain conditions.

On the other hand, if we do not have proper understanding, we can create sickness with improper food combinations. Improper food combinations arise when both foods are very yin or very yang, or otherwise produce a combination of both extremes, which results in extreme yin or extreme yang effects to our physical and mental conditions. It is traditionally known that the following combinations of food are not advisable to maintain our health, although ill effects may not arise every time they are eaten, since toxic effects depend also upon the way of preparation, the volume eaten, and our personal constitution and condition:

—Raw clams (yin) and citrus juice (yin)—toxic effects
—*Azuki* rice (slightly more yang) and glovefish (yin)—toxic effects
—Crucian carp (yin) and mustard greens (yin)—produce hemorrhoids
—Horsemeat (yang) and *jinenjo* (mountain potato) (yang)—produce worms
—Buckwheat (yang) and mud snails (yang)—produce intestinal pain
—Fresh clams (yin) and sugar (yin)—produce toxic effects
—Watermelon (yin) and tempura (oil is yin)—produce diarrhea
—Mushroom (yin) and tempura (yin)—produce diarrhea
—Mushroom (yin) and shortnecked clam (yin)—produce intestinal pain
—Mint (yin) and potato (yin)—produce toxic effects
—Burdock (yang) and trout (yang)—produce intestinal pain
—Octopus (yin) and plums (yin)—produce toxic effects
—Quail (yin) and mushrooms (yin)—produce toxic effects
—Loquat (yin) and *azuki* beans (yin)—produce intestinal pain
—Duck egg (yang) and *jinenjo* (mountain potato) (yang)—produce intestinal pain
—Catfish (yang) and pork (yang)—produce toxic effects
—Leek (yin) and honey (yin)—produce acute pain
—Glovefish (yin) and summer greens (yin)—produce toxic effects
—Crabmeat (yin) and persimmon (yin)—produce toxic effects
—Caviar (yang) and liver (yang)—produce toxic effects
—Buckwheat (yang) and *jijube* (yang)—produce intestinal pain
—Egg (yang) and garlic (yin)—produce toxic effects
—Crabmeat (yin) and ice water (yin)—produce diarrhea
—Bamboo shoots (yin) and sugar (yin)—produce intestinal pain

chapter 5

Human Sicknesses: Cause and Recovery

> We are grateful for all difficulties, sickness,
> poverty, confusion, hardship, and war. Because
> of them, we learn of our own ignorance, inability,
> and dependence. Because of them we strengthen
> ourselves and develop towards freedom. All
> difficulties are caused not by any external
> factors, but by ourselves. Let us enjoy all
> difficulties and let us turn them into happiness.
>
> January, 1977

1. Cause of Difficulties

We, Man, came from the infinite universe, physicalizing and materializing ourselves upon this earth, through hundreds of billions of journeys of life. We all shall continue this journey of life beyond our life as human beings, through dephysicalization and spiritualization towards the infinite universe, our origin. During this long journey, our life as a human being on this planet is fundamentally one of health and well-being without any feeling of difficulty. Because we are a part of the environment and we change according to the change of environment, we are natively harmonious with any circumstance and therefore there should be no difficulty. However, almost everyone, throughout many centuries, has experienced various kinds of difficulty, including the struggle for survival and continuation of life itself. Mankind has experienced difficulties not only through natural catastrophes and geological change, but also, difficulties arising in human behavior: physical, mental, and spiritual sicknesses, social and ideological confusions, are everywhere throughout the world, and even our modern civilization itself is in a state of sickness. Why are we suffering from various sicknesses? Why are we struggling with various difficulties?

All of those difficulties are due to our ignorance of what we are, of what life is, of our relationship with our environment, and of the order of the universe. We may have gained the fruit of the tree of knowledge, but we have not gained the fruit of the tree of life. As far as the problems of life are concerned, we are all hopelessly ignorant. Sciences have developed, technologies have prospered, doctrines have prevailed; theories, assumptions, hypotheses and discoveries have been mounting for the past centuries. Yet, we do not know what life is. In our search for happiness, have we not looked in the wrong direction? Are our modern methods by which we try to solve the problems of life, reaching a dead end? We are proud of our level of education which is higher than that of primitive man. We are proud of our material wealth surpassing the wealth of ancient people. We are proud of our organized

[103]

society which is more universal than in the olden times, and we are proud of our knowledge, more far-reaching than in the prehistoric age. And yet, every one of us is full of fear and anxiety, worry and depression, and surrounded with sickness and violence, greed and hatred, prejudice and insecurity. What is the cause of all this suffering? What is the origin of these troubles? How can we solve these difficulties, and how are we to approach these confusions?

To deal with these problems, we have developed a comprehensive system of education universally available for all modern people. We have developed a remarkable governmental system covering every individual living everywhere. We have built an impressive medical welfare system applying to every person in the present society. Hundreds of billions of dollars are spent, and millions of people are working for these systems to meet the difficulties we are facing at the present time. Are these methods adequate, proper, and sufficiently effective to build our physical, mental and spiritual health? Are these systems really serving towards the solution of our problems? Is there any other method which is simple and practical enough that everyone can practice it in his daily life without any strain? If there is such a method, what is it?

Let us begin by finding the definition of health and well-being.

A. Definition of Health

Health is not the state of being without sickness; it is a more positive and creative state of physical, mental and spiritual life. Health is not something to be secured by defending and preserving ourselves from suffering with disease; rather, it is a state of actively harmonizing with our environment, of enjoying with many other people, of ceaseless creation and progress. Our health should satisfy the following seven conditions:

(1) *Never be tired:* In day-to-day life, we should not feel any fatigue if we are healthy. After a day's work, we should not complain, "I am tired." Whatever hardship we may encounter, we should be able to adapt to it with an energetic desire to work it out. From time to time we may feel exhaustion from our work, but we should recover from it after a short rest or a night's sleep. Not only in our physical condition, but also in our mental affairs, we should not feel tired. If we are fre-

---

Longevity in the Ancient World

"The Yellow Emperor once addressed T'ien Shih, the divinely inspired teacher: "I have heard that in ancient times the people lived (through the years) to be over a hundred years, and yet they remained active and did not become decrepit in their activities. But nowadays people reach only half of their age and yet become decrepit and failing. Is it because the world changes from generation to generation? Or is it that mankind is becoming negligent (of the laws of nature)?"

"Ch'i Po answered: "In ancient times those people who understood Tao (the way of self-cultivation) patterned themselves upon the yin and the yang (the two principles in nature) and they lived in harmony with the arts of divination.

"There was temperance in eating and drinking. Their hours of rising and retiring were regular and not disorderly and wild. By these means the ancients kept their bodies united with their souls, so as to fulfill their allotted span completely, measuring unto a hundred years before they passed away."

Yellow Emperor's Classic of Internal Medicine, Book I, Ch. 1, P. 97, Iliza Veith, Translator.

quently changing our mind, so that we often wish to change our ideas and plans, occupation and address, we are in an unhealthy state. Under any circumstance at any time, we should maintain a physical and mental state able to respond immediately to the changing circumstances, and able to approach the new environment with a spirit of adventure.

(2) *Have Good Appetite:* In our daily life, and throughout our life, we should always have a good appetite for whatever we may encounter. Appetite for food, appetite for sex, appetite for activity, appetite for knowledge, appetite for work, appetite for experience, and appetite for health, freedom and happiness. Endless appetite is a manifestation of health, and limited appetite is a manifestation of sickness. The bigger our appetite is, the richer our life is. Without appetite there is no progress, no development, and no enjoyment of this life. However, in order to keep a large appetite continuously, we should wisely avoid over-satisfaction of the appetite. When we are hungry, we should eat so as to satisfy 80% of our hunger, leaving a portion of the stomach unfilled. Over-satisfaction reduces our appetite and gradually slows down our life activity. Therefore, we should keep ourselves always hungry, and as soon as we take in, we should distribute whatever we have received and keep always emptiness within ourselves.

(3) *Have Good Sleep:* Good sleep is not sleep of long duration, but rather, deep sleep for a shorter time. Good sleep is a result of energetic activity—physical and mental—during the time we are awake. While we are sleeping, we should not experience any sort of dream which we remember after we awake. If we remember a dream after we awake, it is because our sleep is not deep enough. Nightmares, cloudy dreams and fragmental dreams are all signs of our physical and mental unrest. To see these dreams frequently is an indication of the beginning of mental illness. Suppose we are frequently frightened with the horrors of nightmares. We are seeing "daymares" through our same physical and mental quality while we are awake. We bother ourselves with unnecessary suspicions, illusions of horrors, and undefended insecurity. If we eat macrobiotically and develop our health, we will never suffer with rootless dreams of any kind. From time to time, however, we may see a dream that comes true—true dream. When we see no dream or see only a true dream during our sleep, we are seeing real circumstances; and whatever we dream as true dream corresponds to our activities and occurrences of the daytime.[1]

(4) *Have Good Memory:* Memory is the mother of our judgment. Without memory of what we have experienced, we would have no judgment or ability to evaluate the changing circumstances. Good memory is the foundation of all sound mental activities; they all come out of memory and return to memory. There are various kinds of memory: mechanical memory, such as the remembrance of numbers and names; memory of images, such as remembrance of scenery and events;

---

[1] *Saying in the ancient Orient:* "A sage does not see a dream. If he does, it is a true dream." True dream is a dream that also happens in reality. For example, there are some instances of accidents happening after we see them in dreams. In primitive society, a dream at night was considered as reality, and when one saw a dream of some event, he attempted to realize it. After all, life is a dream, whether we are awake or sleeping. As a popular song describes, "Row, row, row your boat, gently down the stream . . . life is but a dream."

and the remembrance of where we have come from and how we have realized ourselves in this world at this time—the memory of spiritual destiny. Among these varieties of memory, the most important is the last, spiritual memory, by which we can understand the significance of our life, and the meaning of the present, and develop our endless appreciation for the past and our limitless aspiration to the future. Good memory is essential to our meaningful life. All other memories, including mechanical memory and memory of images, are actually part of this memory of our spiritual origin and destiny. As we continue to live macrobiotically, we begin to recover not only various memories of daily events, but also this memory of spiritual destiny.[2]

(5) *Never Be Angry:* Throughout our lifetime we should never be angry. Since we are living within the infinite universe and we are all living in harmony with our environment, there is no reason to be angry. We know that everyone, everything and every phenomenon is nothing but complementary to one another—including our enemies. We should never be angry if we are in good health. Being angry shows our limitation, our inability to understand and embrace, our lack of patience and perseverance. The character for "anger" (怒) in Far Easterns countries describes anger as the mind (心) of a slave (奴). Another word for "anger" (肝癪) means acute sickness (癪) of the liver (肝). In oriental medicine, anger is correlated with the sickness of the liver, as other major mental reactions are correlated respectively with sicknesses of other major organs.[3] Those who do not know how to cope with various circumstances become often excited, while those who know how to solve a situation do not feel any anger. Health is to accept all circumstances with a smile and turn our enemy into our friend, change difficulty into our comfort.

(6) *Be Joyous and Alert:* In order to live an active and productive life, it is necessary to respond immediately to the constantly changing environment. Life is a continuous progression of such responses. We should be accurate in our expression, speedy in our motion, orderly in our behavior, and clear in our thinking. These responses to be made moment to moment should be full of joy and humor. Bright optimism and merry thoughts should radiate from our life to everyone else. Greetings should be exchanged actively with people every morning, every evening, and

---

[2] *Mutual Understanding:* It is commonly experienced between two persons and among many people, that they easily understand what each other is trying to say, or that they easily agree with each other, although they may have been born in different places and brought up and educated in different ways. The reason they can understand each other is that they have common universal memory, whether or not they are aware of it. Because of their common background in the origin of their life, because of the oneness in which they were together, they can now understand each other and can say, "Yes, I agree with you." This common origin is nothing but the one infinite universe itself.

[3] *Disease of Organs and Emotions:* In oriental medicine, there has been a traditional understanding that emotional symptoms are the result of sicknesses of certain organs, and certain emotions affect certain organs. The liver and gall bladder correlate with anger and excitement; the heart and small intestine with laughing and talkativeness; the spleen-pancreas and stomach with conceptuality and skepticism; the lungs and large intestine with depression and melancholy; and the kidneys and bladder with fear and insecurity.

whenever meeting on the street. Good morning, good evening, how are you, and thank you, are to be given openly to any other person, with a smile. Joyous life is a natural result of health, and it gives joy and happiness to people surrounding us, like the sun which radiates its light and warmth to every life upon the earth.

(7) *Have Endless Appreciation:* As human beings who are manifestations of the infinite order of the universe, we should know our eternal life, and we should know that everyone and every being who have also come out in the universe, are all brothers and sisters. We should have clear understanding that there is nothing really opposing us and if we feel some difficulties, it is because of our own illusions. Endless appreciation for the order of the universe and for all phenomena manifesting within this universe is the way of life of a person who has health—physically, mentally and spiritually. We are healthy when we are receiving from everything with endless gratitude, and giving of ourselves without hesitation—our ideas, our materials, our activity, our energy, and even our life itself—to all from whom and from which we have received. Even when we are in physical sickness, we are healthy when we are aware that the cause of such sickness is coming from ourselves, and when we are thankful for the opportunity to learn, and submit our destiny to the hand of the order of the universe with endless appreciation.

B. Development of Sickness

All physical, mental, and spiritual sicknesses are closely interrelated and have a similar progressive development—as from a single root, many branches and leaves grow. There is no independent sickness which has a cause and process of development that is separate and unrelated to all other sicknesses and conditions. However numerous the symptomatic appearances may be, and however distinguishable a particular symptom may be from another, they are all connected and related with one another, and their causes are practically the same. In order to find the solution for various problems of sickness, we must search for the real cause underlying these sick symptoms. In modern medical practice, what we usually consider to be the cause of a certain sickness is often only a symptom which develops into a sickness, and not the real cause.

For example, in the case of hypertension (high blood pressure), it is well known that the cause of the condition is the enlargement of the heart or the constriction of blood vessels and capillaries. However, these causes are nothing but physical symp-

---

Anger in Private Affairs and Anger in Public Affairs: There are two kinds of anger: one is called "personal anger" or SHI-FUN (私憤) and another is called "public anger" or KOH-FUN (公憤). Private anger is excitement over personal affairs, often seen among individuals; public anger is anger for social injustice and the sacrifices of many people. Invariably, personal anger is a sign of physical and mental sickness; but public anger is sometimes a result of conscience. If we are in truly good health, however, even social injustice which may be producing public suffering, should not cause us to react in anger. Instead, such injustices should be appreciated as the opportunity to make people learn and strengthen themselves, and should be turned into happiness for everyone. We can discover the cause of the injustice and find a solution that is peaceful—not by revolutionary violence, but through biological change of human thought. Even the way of nonviolence or passive resistance which mobilizes massive power, is a method inferior to the biological change of human nature.

toms which lead to high blood pressure. What is the real cause, which is producing these conditions of heart enlargement and constriction of the blood vessels and capillaries? Let us look at another example: physical and mental fatigue caused by an anemic condition, due to a lack of iron, other minerals, or certain vitamins. In the symptomatic approach to this sickness, one attempts to supply the missing minerals and vitamins in the form of capsules, injections, special food supplements and similar measures. This approach would relieve the symptoms of anemia temporarily, but it would not prevent the recurrence of the symptoms unless there were a basic change in daily dietary habits.

All sicknesses—physical, mental, and spiritual—have four factors in their development:

(1) *Symptoms:* These are what we usually call sickness or disease, and explicitly appear as uncomfortable, abnormal expressions—pain, itching, fever, coughing, vomiting, etc.

(2) *Conditions:* The various symptoms are produced by underlying conditions. For example, as discussed above, the symptom of hypertension is produced by the underlying condition of enlargement of the heart and constriction of the blood vessels and capillaries.

(3) *Cause:* Every condition, which is producing various symptoms, has a cause, which is found in various aspects of our physical and mental tendencies, especially the general quality of our blood.

(4) *Origin:* These causes of sicknesses—our general physical and mental tendencies, particularly our blood quality—originate in our daily habits, including dietary practice, physical exercise, mental activity, and our general view of life. In other words, all sicknesses have their origin in our way of life viewed as a whole.

Accordingly, there are three categories of medicine:

(1) *Symptomatic and conditional medicine,* which has been commonly practiced in modern western medicine, and which includes trying to eliminate symptoms or change conditions by the use of various technical measures, such as the performance of surgery and the use of pharmaceutical medications.

(2) *Medicine for the cause,* which deals mainly with the problem of blood and energy change through the change of what we consume in the form of food and drink; including various kinds of dietary practices with vitamin and mineral supple-

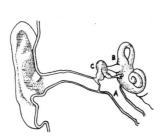

Increase in Deafness and Difficulty of Hearing
In modern civilized society, deafness and difficulty of hearing are rapidly increasing due to accumulated fat and mucus in the region of the inner ear (A) which may even spread within the region of the cochlea (B). It also makes the transmitting bones (C) stick together. Deafness and hearing difficulties are also caused by the loss of sensitivity of the audial nerves, either by the expansion of the nerve cells or by the congealing of liquid within the cochlea (B). The first condition occurs because of excessive intake of animal fat, dairy food, and sugar. The second condition is caused by the excessive intake of sugar-treated icy soft drinks, cold food such as ice cream, spices, and other stimulants, as well as excessive intake of liquid and dairy food.

ments, herbal remedies, and various physical and mental adjustments and exercises.

(3) *Medicine by the way of life*, which is more philosophical and educational rather than technical and artificial, and which attempts to recover the proper way of life based upon self-reflection, through the understanding of the relation between man and his environment, as well as the order of nature and of the universe.

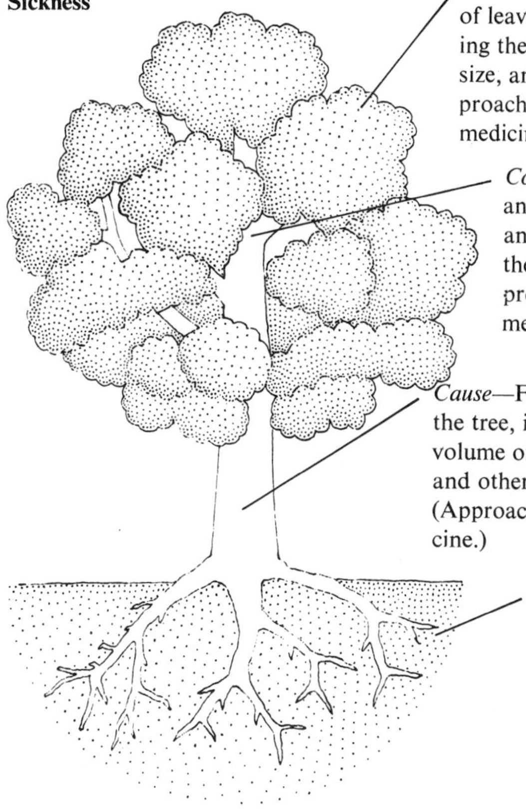

Fig. 31 The Tree of Sickness

Symptoms—Various symptoms of disorders manifesting physically and mentally.

Conditions—General disharmony of cells, tissues, organs, and systems.

Cause—Wrong dietary habits and degraded quality of blood and body fluid.

Origin—Lack of understanding of the order of the universe; wrong way of life, out of harmony with nature.

Symptoms—Appearances of leaves and stems, including their color, texture, size, and activities (approached by symptomatic medicine).

Conditions—Structure and quality of tissues and cells as well as their functioning. (Approached by adjustment of conditions.)

Cause—Fluid streaming within the tree, including quality and volume of water, minerals, and other nutritional contents. (Approached by dietary medicine.)

Origin—Environment, including climate, weather, water, soil, and other natural conditions. (Approached by environmental medicine.)

The Attitude of Oriental Medicine: Oriental medicine practiced in China, India, Japan and other Asian countries from a time unknown ages ago, possibly about 5,000 years ago, until the beginning of widespread westernization about 100 years ago, has as its primary approach, either medicine for the cause or medicine by the way of life. It classifies the kinds of medicine into three:

Highest medicine— Treatment of the whole personality and way of life, mainly through general guidance towards self-reflection and self-improvement of daily life.

Middle medicine— Treatment of cause, mainly through dietary change, physical exercise, and adjustment of energy flow.

Lower medicine— Symptomatic treatment, mainly through medicinal and surgical practice.

It also classifies into three the doctors who deal with sicknesses:

Highest doctors— Those who treat and heal various sicknesses of society, the country, and the world through philosophy and education about the proper way of life.

Middle doctors— Those who treat and heal a person who is suffering with sickness, through changing his personal habits.

Lower doctors— Those who treat and heal sicknesses symptomatically but who do not treat the whole personality of the patient.

All physical, mental and spiritual sicknesses have their origins in our daily life. If our daily way of living is not in harmony with our environment and does not enable us to maintain our status as human beings, biologically and psychologically, in the changing atmosphere on the present earth, we are compelled to adjust to the environment by unusual methods which appear as various symptoms of sicknesses, or to change ourselves through a process of gradual degeneration. All sicknesses, therefore, can be classified into two large categories: *adjustment* and *degeneration*.

Sicknesses of adjustment usually appear as acute symptoms, and after our harmonious relation with the environment has been recovered, the symptoms disappear. These sicknesses include various types of fever, coughing, diarrhea, skin disease, aches and pains, as well as emotional symptoms—irritability, nervousness, depression and excitement. On the other hand, *degenerative sicknesses* usually appear in the form of chronic suffering, and their degenerative tendency progressively deepens and widens unless the course of degeneration is reversed toward the recovery of our human qualities by the establishment of harmonious relations between ourselves and our environment.

Generally speaking, our sicknesses take the following progressive pattern in their development:

1st Stage—General Fatigue: A feeling of physical and mental tiredness is the beginning of sickness. This condition is often accompanied by muscular tension and hardening, frequent urination and sweating, temporary constipation or diarrhea, and short periods of feeling cold or hot. Mentally, we start to lose our clarity of thought, active perception and accurate responses. In order to recover from this stage, it takes usually a short period—from a few hours to a few days—by taking rest, overnight sleep, proper food and drink, or adequate exercise.

2nd Stage—Aches and Pains: When a feeling of general fatigue becomes our usual state, we begin to have occasional pains and aches. Muscular pain, headache, cramps, and various other sorts of pains and aches appear here and there. Temporary shortness of breath, irregular heartbeat, fever and chills, and difficulty of motion also appear in this stage. Mentally, we may experience occasional depression, worry, and a general feeling of insecurity. To restore ourselves to health from this stage usually takes a few days to a few weeks, with proper dietary practice, active exercise, or necessary rest.

3rd Stage—Blood Disease: If our dietary practice continues out of balance with our environment, our quality of blood, including red blood cells, white blood cells, and blood plasma becomes unsuitable for maintaining a harmonious relation with our natural surroundings. Blood further changes into our cells, and therefore the quality of the cells and tissues of various parts of the body develops an abnormal condition, from which various sick symptoms arise. Acidosis, high and low blood pressure, anemia, purpura, leukemia, scurvy, and other sicknesses belong to this stage, including asthma, epilepsy, and skin diseases. Mentally, this stage appears as nervousness, hypersensitivity, continuous depression, timidity, and loss of general direction. To recover from these blood diseases may take between ten days and a few months, by changing the previous diet to conform to proper practices, with suitable exercise and rest. Simple treatment to promote active circulation of the blood may be required in some cases.

4th Stage—Emotional Disorder: If an improper quality of blood circulates for a prolonged period, various emotional disorders start to arise frequently. Short temper, excitement, anger, frustration, and a general feeling of despair are experienced in daily life. A gentle approach to a problem with objective understanding becomes no longer possible. A general feeling of fear prevails in the attitude toward unaccustomed situations, and unnecessary expressions—either defensive or offensive—appear often in daily behavior. Physical movement becomes also more rigid with a gradual loss of flexibility. It requires between one month and several months to overcome these emotional and physical disorders. Dietary change towards more balanced food is essential, along with physical and mental relaxation.

5th Stage—Organ Disease: An imbalanced quality of blood circulating for a prolonged period further produces gradual changes of the organs and glands in their quality and function. Structural change, malfunction and degeneration start to arise. Arteriosclerosis, diabetes, stone formation in the kidneys and gall bladder, various sorts of cancer, multiple sclerosis and many other sicknesses are in this category. Mentally, chronic stubbornness, prejudice, narrow-mindedness, and general rigidity with an illusional interpretation of circumstances become more apparent. To recover from this level of disease, it generally takes a longer period, several months to one year, by the continuous practice of proper diet and the change of the way of life, with self-reflection.

6th Stage—Nervous Disorder: From the stage of organ and gland disease, the degenerative tendency deepens toward various nervous disorders including physical paralysis and mental illnesses such as schizophrenia and paranoia. Physical and mental coordination in various functions progressively diminishes. A negative view begins to dominate daily life, and suicidal or destructive delusions frequently manifest. It would take six months to a few years to recover completely from this stage, and to regain self-assurance and trust as well as a positive view of life. The way of

---

Antagonistic-Complemental Relations, Yin and Yang, Among Major Organs

Organ	Structure	Electromagnetic (Ki) Flow in Meridian
Group I		
Liver	Yang (△)	Yin (△)
Gall bladder	Yin (▽)	Yang (▽)
Group II		
Heart	Yang (△)	Yin (△)
Small intestine	Yin (▽)	Yang (▽)
Group III		
Spleen and pancreas	Yang (△)	Yin (△)
Stomach	Yin (▽)	Yang (▽)
Group IV		
Lungs	Yang (△)	Yin (△)
Large intestine	Yin (▽)	Yang (▽)
Group V		
Kidney	Yang (△)	Yin (△)
Bladder	Yin (▽)	Yang (▽)

life has to be changed completely, including dietary practice, more harmonious relationship with the environment, and active physical exercise, together with loving care by the surrounding people.

7th Stage—Arrogance: An improper way of life which has been practiced for many years finally reaches the highest level of sickness, arrogance, although some of the previous stages may not have been clearly experienced. Arrogance is the most developed sickness, and also the one which most universally affects people's lives. Selfishness, egocentricity, vanity, self-pride, exclusivity and self-justification are some of the common symptoms. Arrogance is the last stage of sickness and at the same time, it is the cause of all other sickness, misery, and unhappiness. Because of the arrogance which has prevailed among many populations, the entire world is full of sickness, not only physically and mentally, but also socially and ideologically. In order to cure this sickness, it takes from a few years to an indefinite length of time, by the practice of the proper way of life. However, arrogance can also be cured instantaneously if unusual emotional or spiritual stimulation is experienced, usually in occasions of difficulties and failure. Cure of arrogance immediately produces a spirit of humility and modesty. It restores also the spirit of appreciation through the self-discovery of our ignorance. When it happens, new life begins with the automatic practice of the way of life in harmony with the environment.

Every physical, mental and spiritual sickness belongs in one of the seven levels outlined above. All sicknesses are interdependent and interconnected with one another; they are symptoms branching out from the same root—improper way of life. Because man is fundamentally nothing but a natural manifestation which has appeared on this earth according to the evolving order of the universe, it is a simple matter to remain in that state of natural order and harmony, and it is more complicated and difficult to develop and suffer from various sicknesses. Modern people, however, are suffering with many sicknesses—and an increasing number of them are degenerative diseases. It has become a common belief that man frequently suffers with some sort of sicknesses and that he must eventually die because of them. This universal belief in modern society is contradictory to the real nature of humanity. As long as man follows and lives with the laws of nature, the order of the universe, as he has been oriented from the beginning, he is able to enjoy his health, and he would rarely suffer from any sort of sickness.

C. Kinds of Human Death

Our human death is, simply speaking, nothing other than suicide. We human beings, because of our potentially free consciousness and free ability to change ourselves, are choosing our own destinies, whether we are aware of it or not. When, how, and where we are going to die are being determined by various accumulated factors—physical and mental, spiritual and social—which we are causing ourselves to experience through our own way of life. Let us consider the various modes of death:

(1) *Biological Death:* If our daily lives, including our dietary practices, are out of harmony with the changing natural environment, our physical and mental conditions become unsuitable for the continuation of our life. This sort of death comes

through various physical and mental sicknesses. In modern society, the majority of deaths belong to this category.

(2) *Psychological Death:* As a result of the continuous practice of an improper way of life, our mentality—which normally appreciates and finds entertainment in our surroundings, natural and social—becomes incapable of seeing the possible happiness of living as human beings. We start to produce psychological delusions, motivating the early termination of our human life. This death appears as committing suicide, or as simply giving up the will to live, usually during a period in which we are experiencing difficulties and pressure. This kind of death is seen in modern society less frequently than biological death, but is increasing throughout the world, even among younger generations.

(3) *Social Death:* In modern societies which have been organized according to a conceptual image, often unconnected to real, natural conditions, we are educated to serve and give our lives for a social cause of some kind, which is often unrelated to the more natural human consciousness. Because of such conceptual beliefs, we participate in groups which are to be killed on the battlefields of civil or foreign wars. Often, millions of human lives are involved in massive destruction with carefully justified methods of warfare. Some millions of people are taking this course of death in every century.

(4) *Accidental Death:* Deaths caused by accidents are increasing continuously in the modern world. It is a common belief that accidents are unavoidable, and that therefore, unexpected misfortune is inescapable. However, accidents are experienced when our physical, mental, and spiritual conditions become unclear as a result of an unhealthy way of life. Our lack of foresight and sensitivity, our carelessness and overexcitement, our lack of clear judgment, are the major causes of accidents and accidental deaths. Whether we are the active creator of an accident or the passive recipient, it is our inadequate ability to continue our life which is the cause of such death.

(5) *Ideological Death:* There are some people who die with clear and stable minds. This kind of death is a meaningful measure, to express deep apologies, taking responsibility for what we have done to others or to the general public. Self-termination of human life has been seen here and there in history. In some cases, death is initiated to encourage and inspire the remaining people and the younger generations. In other cases, we continue to pursue our dream, although we know that we shall have to meet unnatural death in the course of such pursuit.[4]

(6) *Natural Death:* When we live according to the order of nature, with continuous practice of proper diet and active physical and mental work in harmonious relationship with other people and society, our lives become prolonged more than

---

[4] *Examples of Ideological Death:* (A) Over a period of nearly ten years in connection with the war in Vietnam, on several occasions groups of peaceloving Buddhist monks burned themselves in an attempt to inspire deep reflection in the remaining people. (B) Traditionally, among Japanese *samurai*, self-termination of life was done in the form of *seppuku* (切腹)—*harakiri*—to take responsibility for their conduct or to honor their country, laws, or traditions. Even in the modern age at the end of World War II, there were many incidences of *harakiri* among military and civil leaders.

the average. In such cases, we die as trees that wither in a change of climate. We feel clearly when and how our death would come. Such death arises very naturally without any particular suffering, and clarity of consciousness remains until the actual death takes place. These kinds of death were often experienced among older people, even two and three generations ago. These elders were full of widsom and were often guiding many young people. They often chose the way, time and place of their death, and after they passed away, their families or other intimate friends would often find arrangements that they had made in preparation for their death. Natural death is characterized by the dying elders' acceptance of death as a natural process, with deep appreciation of life itself.[5]

(7) *Spiritual Death:* On rare occasions, death as a means of further evolution from human status to the spiritual world is experienced among spiritually-developed people. Often such death is self-initiated, and such a person often disappears by his own will, perhaps to the mountains or to the wilderness where he wishes to end his life. In other cases, he may dissolve his body in front of his friends, or elevate himself towards the atmospheric vibrational world.[6]

With the exception of massive death arising by natural catastrophes, all human deaths belong to one of the above categories. Among modern people, death is most often of the biological, psychological, social and accidental varieties rather than ideological, natural and spiritual. The former are kinds of death resulting from physical, mental and spiritual sickness, and the latter are from a healthy life conducted in the macrobiotic order. The macrobiotic way of life leads to not only the improvement of our physical and mental health, but also to the development of our spiritual ability towards the self-elevation of our life to the further world.

---

[5] *Natural Death and Instinct:* Except in occasions of natural catastrophe and interference by man and other species, wild animals generally experience natural death. They know the time of their death before it comes. It is well known that wild elephants travel to the depths of the jungle towards their natural cemeteries when they feel that death is coming. Even among domesticated animals this instinct remains. Cats and dogs hide their bodies when they are going to die, if circumstances allow; rats that live aboard ships often escape while the boats are in port, knowing that the coming voyage may meet with severe storm or fire. Such instinct is natively working in all species, including our human race, if we are following the order of nature.

[6] *Examples of Spiritual Death:*

A. Lao Tzu (老子), 5th century B.C., a philosopher in China, is known to have disappeared after riding a donkey out of the gate of the country—KANKOKU-KAN (函谷関), and no one knows how he ended his life. Just before he left, he wrote articles setting forth his understanding of the order of the universe, which became a small book, the TAO TEH CHING (道徳経).

B. Elias (8th century B.C.), a prophet in Israel, also experienced a spiritual death, as we see in the following passage from the Bible: "And when they were gone over, Elias said to Eliseus: Ask what thou wilt have me do for thee, before I be taken away from thee. And Eliseus said: I beseech thee that in me may be thy double spirit. And he answered: Thou hast asked a hard thing: nevertheless if thou see me when I am taken from thee, thou shalt have what thou hast asked: but if thou see me not, thou shalt not have it. And as they went on, walking and talking together, behold a fiery chariot, and fiery horses parted both asunder: and Elias went up by a whirlwind into heaven." (IV Kings 2:9–11).

2. Yin and Yang in Physical and Mental Sicknesses

All physical and mental sicknesses can be classified according to their symptoms and causes into three major categories: (1) those caused by excessive yin—centrifugal and expansive tendency; (2) those caused by excessive yang—centripetal and contractive tendency; and (3) those caused by both excessive yin and excessive yang.

The following tables show examples of symptoms and diseases, arranged according to these three major categories.

Examples of Yin and Yang Disorders

Disorders of the Skin and Hair		
Yin ($\triangledown$)	Yang ($\triangle$)	Yin($\triangledown$) and Yang($\triangle$) Combined
Representative Symptoms:		
Increased redness	Bluish or yellowish (jaundiced) appearance	Hardening and thickening of the skin
Inflammation, swelling	Constriction of capillaries	Tumor with pus discharge
Watery discharge	Dryness of surface skin	
Disintegration of tissue		
Diseases:		
Allergy	Asphyxiation	Skin Cancer
Infection	Pallor	Pigmentation, as in Addison's disease
Fever	Cyanosis by incomplete oxygenation of blood	
Hyperemia		Warts, moles
Baldness—peripheral regions of head	Baldness—central regions of head	Baldness—complete
Freckles	Grey hair	White patches
Extreme moisture resulting from hyperthyroidism	Extreme dryness as in heat stroke	
Hypertension		Elephantitis
Emotional disturbance		

Smoking and Lung Cancer

It is currently well known that smoking is causing the development of lung cancer among the people of modern society who consume excessive quantities of saturated fat and other fatty acids as well as mucus-forming food, together with sugar and sugar-treated food and stimulant beverages. This is statistically proven. However, among the populations who do not consume these foods but who consume more unrefined grains, vegetables, beans, and seaweed, or who consume food according to traditional practices, the development of lung cancer due to smoking is not statistically proven.

The foundation to develop lung cancer is the quality of the blood which produces potential cancer cells in the lungs, together with the accumulation of mucus in the alveoli (air sacs). With this basis, smoking can work as a stimulant agent to produce cancer. In other words, for those who do not consume an excessive volume of animal food, including meat, eggs, and dairy food, as well as refined sugar, honey, tropical and semi-tropical fruits, fruit juices, wine and other alcoholic beverages, and various stimulant aromatic beverages, smoking does not contribute to produce lung cancer. It is, however, not advisable to smoke heavily—for many other physical, mental, and economic reasons—especially for women and children.

Disorders of the Muscular System

Yin (▽)	Yang (△)	Yin(▽) and Yang(△) Combined
Representative Symptoms:		
Sudden paralysis	Gradual paralysis	Immobility
Swelling	Constriction	Constriction
Inflammation	Hardening	Inflammation
General weakness		General weakness
Pains		
Tension	Immobility	
Diseases:		
Tetany	Tetanus (lockjaw)	Stiffness of neck and shoulder
Cramp		
"Charley-horse"	Sprain	Torticollis (wryneck)
Hernia		
Spasm		
Progressive muscular dystrophy	Myotonia	Muscular atrophy
		Myositis
		Myasthenia gravis

Disorders in Blood and Body Fluids

Yin (▽)	Yang (△)	Yin(▽) and Yang(△) Combined
Representative Symptoms:		
Lack of vitality	General fatigue	General fatigue
General fatigue		
Dilation, swelling, inflammation	Constriction of circulatory vessels	Hardening
Reduction of red blood cells	Reduction of white blood cells, in some cases	Imbalance among blood cell number
Bleeding	Thickening of blood	Higher cholesterol and fatty content in blood
Weakening of arterial and venous walls	Bleeding	
Diseases:		
Nutritional anemia	Scurvy	Pernicious anemia
Hemophilia		
Leukemia		Hodgkins' disease
Purpura		Lymphosarcoma
Coronary occlusion		Hypertension (high blood pressure)
Angina pectoris	Some hardening of arteries	
Hypertension (high blood pressure)		Hypotension (low blood pressure)
Hypotension (low blood pressure)		Arteriosclerosis
Irregular heartbeat		Atherosclerosis
Heart block		Some hardening of arteries
Phlebitis		
Varicose veins		
Variocele		
Fibrillation		
Some cases of fluttering	Some cases of fluttering	
Tachycardia	Bradycardia	

Disorders of the Bones and Joints

Yin (▽)	Yang (△)	Yin(▽) and Yang(△) Combined
Representative Symptoms:		
Swelling	Consolidation of joints	Swelling
Inflammation	Abnormal inward curve and	Inflammation
Softening or deformation	deformation	Stiffness and deformation
Infectious conditions	Immobility	Hardening
Diseases:		
Some cancers, such as bone cancer	Some cancers, such as joint cancer	Some cancers, such as bone marrow cancer
Infectious arthritis	Metabolic arthritis—(gout)	Rheumatoid arthritis
Osteoarthritis		Bursitis
Osteomyelitis	Osteitis fibrosa	
Osteomalacia		
Bunion		
Flat foot	Club foot	
Acromegaly	Hunchback	
Frequent dislocation		
Rickets		Paget's disease
Pott's disease		
Scoliosis		

Disorders of the Digestive System

Yin (▽)	Yang (△)	Yin(▽) and Yang(△) Combined
Representative Symptoms:		
Swelling	Constriction; sometimes swelling	Swelling
Inflammation	Inflammation	Inflammation
Looseness of tissue	Hardening	
Enlargement of organs	Formation of pus and tumors	Production of pus and tumors
Spasmic pains		Lack of metabolic coordination
Slowness of metabolism	Fever	
Diseases:		
Tooth decay	Tooth erosion	
Inflammation of gums		
Chronic constipation and diarrhea	Temporary constipation	Obesity
Vomiting	Diarrhea	
Some cancer such as stomach, colon, and esophagus cancer	Some cancer such as liver, duodenum, and rectum cancer	Some cancer such as pancreatic cancer
Mumps	Appendicitis	Hemerrhoids
Adenoids	Cholecystis	
Tonsilitis		
Colitis		
Gastric pancreatitis		
Stomach ulcers	Duodenal ulcers	
Cirrhosis	Jaundice	Hepatitis
Dysentery		Cholera
Diabetes		Typhoid fever
Harelip		Gallstones

Disorders of the Respiratory System

Yin (▽)	Yang (△)	Yin(▽) and Yang(△) Combined
Representative Symptoms:		
Dilation of organs and tissues	Constriction of respiratory system	Expansion or constriction in respiratory organs
Difficulty in breathing	Difficulty in breathing	Difficulty in breathing
Inflammation; swelling	Inflammation in some cases	Inflammation in some cases
Infectious conditions		
Diseases:		
Asthma	Shortness of breath	Pneumonia
Bronchitis	Choking	
Croup		Mucus—fat accumulation in lungs
Diphtheria		Empyema
Emphysema		
Hay fever		
Pleurisy		
Tonsilitis		
Adenoids		
Tuberculosis		
Whooping cough		
Some conditions of cyanosis	Some conditions of cyanosis	
Collapsed lung		Consolidation
Some cancer such as throat cancer	Some cancer such as tongue cancer	Lung cancer
Sneezing, hiccoughing		
Yawning, snoring		
Sighing, crying, sobbing		
Some coughing	Some coughing	Some coughing
Stuttering		Gutteral voice

Disorders of the Nervous System

Yin (▽)	Yang (△)	Yin(▽) and Yang(△) Combined
Representative Symptoms:		
Swelling	Constriction and hardening of nervous system	Some expansion and some constriction of nervous system
Inflammation	Inflammation in some cases	
Nervousness		
Trembling		
Numbness	Cold body temperature	
Pain	Sweating	
Watery discharge	Rigidity	Imbalance and instability
Less movement	Greater movement	Accumulation of mucus and fat
Diseases:		
Mental depression	Mental depression	Insecurity
Schizophrenia	Psychopathy	Emotional imbalance
Fear	Paranoia	
Worry	Short temper; anger	
Some frustration	Some frustration	General frustration
Some excitability	Some excitability	
Hypersensitivity	Hate; stubbornness	Resentment
	Narrow view	

Yin (▽)	Yang (△)	Yin(▽) and Yang(△) Combined
Detachment of retina glaucoma		Astigmatism
Some myopia (nearsightedness)	Some myopia (farsightedness)	
Stye		Cataract
Conjunctivitis		
Some color blindness	Some color blindness	
Crossed eyes—outward	Crossed eyes—inward	
Bloodshot eyes		
Transmission and peripheral deafness		Central deafness
Loss of equilibrium		Loss of equilibrium
Some headache—front and more peripheral regions of head	Some headache—deep and at more central and back regions of head	Cauliflower ear
Some Parkinson's disease—small trembling	Some Parkinson's disease—greater shaking	
Some multiple sclerosis	Some multiple sclerosis	
Epilepsy	Grinding teeth	
Meningitis		
Vertigo, dizziness		
Sensation of fatigue	Sensation of hunger	
Loss of memory		
Insomnia	Some Insomnia	
Fragmented dreams	Sleepwalking	Nightmares

Disorders of the Urinary System

Yin (▽)	Yang (△)	Yin(▽) and Yang(△) Combined
Representative Symptoms:		
Swelling	Swelling, especially on joints	Swelling
Water intoxication		
Sweating	Water retention	Sweating
Colorless urine	Sweating	
Expansion of urinary systems	Dark urine	
	Constriction of urinary passages	Constriction or expansion of urinary system
General fatigue	Urination difficulty	Accumulation of mucus and fat in organs
Frequent urination		
Pains and inflammation in some cases		
Diseases:		
Cystitis	Oliguria	Uremia
Enuresis	Dysuria	
Pyelitis		Nephritis
Movable kidney		
Some cancer such as in the bladder	Some cancer	Some cancer such as in kidneys
Some retention	Some retention	Edema
Some anuria	Some stricture	Some anuria
Movable kidney		Kidney stone
Incontinence	Some Bedwetting	
Some Bedwetting	Some Bedwetting	

Disorders of the Endocrine System

Yin (▽)	Yang (△)	Yin(▽) and Yang(△) Combined
Representative Symptoms:		
Hypersecretion of yin hormones, and	Hyposecretion of yin hormones, and	Irregular and unbalanced secretion of yin and yang hormones
Hyposecretion of yang hormones	Hypersecretion of yang hormones	
Expansion in growth	Constriction in growth	Unbalanced growth
General fatigue	General irritability	General frustration
Diseases:		
Exothalmic goiter (Graves' disease)	Simple goiter	Unbalanced and complex yin and yang symptoms combined
Toxic goiter		
Acromegaly	Myxedema (Gull's disease)	Irregular growth
Gigantism		
	Dwarfism	
Pituitary basophilism	Pituitary cachexia (Simmond's disease)	
Diabetes mellitus	Diabetes insipidus	
Tetany	Hyperinsulinism	Dysinsulinism
Addison's disease	Osteitis fibrosa	
	Cushing's syndrome	
	Adrenogenital syndrome	
Hyposecretion of the testes	Sexual precocity	Irregular menstruation
	Virilism	
Hypogonadism	Lack of sexual libido	Frequent change of sexual and physical vitalities
Some menstrual disorders, irregularity	Some menstrual disorders, irregularity	

Disorders of the Reproductive System

Yin (▽)	Yang (△)	Yin(▽) and Yang(△) Combined
Representative Symptoms:		
Disorder and malfunction mainly in male organs	Disorder and malfunction mainly in female organs	Disorder and malfunction in the organs of both sexes
Inflammation, excessive moisture, swelling	More dryness, inflammation and swelling in some cases	Inflammation and swelling in some cases
Loss of sexual libido	Excessive sexual libido	Irregular sexual libido
Diseases:		
Hydrocile	Anorchidism	Breast cysts
Prostatic hypertrophy	Cryptorchism	
	Monorchidism	Chancroid
Some urethral stricture	Some urethral stricture	
Vesculitis	Phimosis	
Retroversion of uterus	Anteversion of uterus	
Prolapsed uterus		Syphilis
Gonorrhea	Vaginismus	Vaginal discharge
Longer menstrual cycle	Shorter menstrual cycle	Irregular menstrual cycle
Some cancer, such as in uterus	Some cancer, such as in vaginal region	Some cancer, such as in prostate and breast regions
Some tumors	Some tumors	Some tumors

3. Approach to Sicknesses

A. General Approach

When the symptoms manifested are generally yin, the approach to the sickness should be to eliminate the causes which produce such yin tendencies, and to make conditions more yang. Likewise, when the symptoms manifested are more yang, the approach should be to change the conditions toward more yin. When the symptoms manifested are both yin and yang, the approach should be to bring the conditions to a middle state, in harmony with the environment.

The adjustments to be made include changes in several aspects of daily living, in the following ways:

(1) *Adjustment of Atmospheric Conditions:* For yin diseases, it is generally advisable to keep the humidity of the surrounding air lower than in the case of other diseases, and to have more sunshine and brightness as well as smooth circulation of air in the room. For yang diseases, it is often advisable to keep the surroundings slightly more moist, dimmer, and with less circulation of air. If the conditions of the disease are both yin and yang combined, the surroundings should generally be kept in a standard condition.

(2) *Adjustment of Activity:* For yin diseases, more active physical exercise is generally advisable, except in cases of pains, fever, fatigue, and exhaustion, all of which, of course, require rest. For yang diseases, on the other hand, it is generally advisable to have less active physical exercise. For diseases of both yin and yang combined, average activity is advisable. Also, for chronic yin diseases, more physical activity is recommended, and for chronic yang diseases, more mental activity.

(3) *Change of Climate:* For a yin disease arising in a colder region or in the winter season, it is often useful to move to a warmer, sunnier climate; while for a yang disease arising in a warmer region or in the summertime, it is often helpful to move to a colder and more northern region. The change of living place is effective because of the natural change of dietary habits which occurs under different climatic conditions.

Adjustment of Environment and Activity		
For Yin(∇) Disease	For Yang($\triangle$) Disease	For Disease Caused by Both Yin and Yang Combined
Atmospheric Condition Should Be:		
Drier	More moist	
Sunnier	Less sunny	General, standard conditions
Brighter light	Dimmer light	
Fresh, cool air	Less air circulation	
Activity Should Be:		
More active, physical exercise	Less active physically	Average activity
Less mental activity	More mental activity	
Climate Should Be:		
Warmer	Colder	Average
Sunnier regions	More northern regions	Normal regions

(4) *Change of Dietary Practices:*   Dietary practices should be changed according to the nature of the causes and symptoms of the diseases—whether yin, yang, or a combination of both. The selection, preparation, and manner of eating of the foods should be carefully managed in order to restore our physical, mental, and spiritual conditions to a state more in harmony with our environment. Such dietary adjustments are to be made according to the following general guidelines for temperate climatic regions:

General Guidelines for Dietary Adjustment		
For Yin($\triangledown$) Diseases	For Yang($\triangle$) Diseases	For Diseases Caused by Both Yin and Yang Combined
Whole Cereal Grains:		
50%–70% of meal	40%–60% of meal	50%–60% of meal
Grains growing in same or colder climatic region	Grains growing in same or warmer climatic region	Grains growing mainly in same climatic region
Beans:		
5%–10% of meal	5%–10% of meal	5%–10% of meal
Smaller, rounder beans growing in same or colder climatic regions, such as *azuki* beans, chickpeas, and lentils	Any beans growing in same or warmer climatic regions	Beans growing mainly in same climatic region
Soup:		
5% of meal	5% of meal	5% of meal
Slightly more *miso, tamari* soy sauce, or sea salt. Slightly saltier and thicker taste. Longer cooking.	Slightly less *miso, tamari* soy sauce, or sea salt. Lighter and less salty taste. Shorter cooking.	Moderate amount of *miso, tamari* soy sauce, or sea salt. A mild salty taste. Moderate amount of cooking.
Vegetables:		
15%–25% of meal	15%–25% of meal	15%–25% of meal
More root and ground vegetables with some leafy vegetables. Longer cooking (10–15 minutes). Slightly more salty seasoning.	More leafy and ground vegetables with less root vegetables. Shorter cooking (2–10 minutes). Slightly less salty seasoning.	More ground vegetables with some leafy and root vegetables. Moderate cooking (5–10 minutes). Moderately salty seasoning.
Animal Food:		
0%–10% of meal	0%–5% of meal	0%–10% of meal
Less or no meat, eggs, poultry, and dairy food. Moderate volume of fish and seafood.	No meat, eggs, poultry and less or no dairy food. Small volume of fish and seafood only when desired.	Less or no meat, eggs, poultry and dairy food. Moderate volume of fish and seafood.
Seaweed:		
5% of meal	5% of meal	5% of meal
Longer cooking	Shorter cooking	Moderate cooking
Thicker taste	Lighter taste	Medium taste
(*Hijiki, arame, kombu* and others)	(*Wakame, nori,* dulse and others)	(Almost any kind)
Salad:		
0%–5% of meal	5% of meal	5% of meal

For Yin(∇) Diseases	For Yang($\triangle$) Diseases	For Diseases Caused by Both Yin and Yang Combined
Primarily none, or occasional use, preferably boiled for 1–3 minutes.	Frequent addition of raw salad vegetables, up to 10% of meal.	Occasional addition of raw salad vegetables.
Seasoning: Sea Salt, Miso, Tamari Soy Sauce:		
Moderate use	Minimum use	Temperate use
Seasoning—Oil:		
Sesame oil, corn oil	Any vegetable oil including olive oil	Sesame, corn, safflower and soybean oils
Minimum use	Moderate use	Mild use
Condiments: Gomasio (Sesame Salt):		
Proportion of roasted sea salt to roasted sesame seeds:	Proportion of roasted sea salt to roasted sesame seeds:	Proportion of roasted sea salt to roasted sesame seeds:
1:8 to 1:10	1:10 to 1:14	1:10 to 1:12
Moderate daily use	Moderate daily use	Moderate daily use
Condiments: Umeboshi, Tekka, Kelp Powder or Other Seaweed Powder:		
Daily use	Occasional use	Frequent use
Moderate volume	Small volume	Moderate volume
Desserts and Snacks:		
Roasted seeds	Roasted seeds	Roasted seeds
No nuts	Roasted nuts in small volume	Roasted nuts in small volume
Generally no fruits, but if craved, occasionally a small volume of dried or cooked fruit	Moderate use of dried, cooked, and fresh local, seasonal fruits	Occasional use of dried, cooked or fresh local, seasonal fruits
Beverage:		
Bancha twig tea	*Bancha* twig tea	*Bancha* twig tea
Mu tea	Light *Mu* tea	Medium *Mu* tea
Cereal grain coffee	Light cereal grain coffee	Medium cereal grain coffee
Herb tea	Light herb tea	Medium herb tea

Although the above outline of daily dietary practices is effective for all sicknesses—physical, mental, and spiritual, there are several points which should be carefully considered:

(*a*) *Cooking:* Even though all foods chosen are non-chemicalized, non-artificial, natural-organic foods, if the way of cooking is not proper, the expected results are not produced. Over- or under-heating, excessive or insufficient use of water, oil, and seasonings, too long or too short time of cooking as well as the use of improper cooking utensils, diminish the beneficial effects of the food. The art of cooking is one of the most important aspects in the healing of various sicknesses, and it requires not only the technical management of cooking, but also a loving spirit on the part of the cook, and a spirit of appreciation in the person who eats.

(*b*) *Volume:* However good the food and the cooking are, their effectiveness is eclipsed by overeating. It is an important practice to avoid overeating and to stop eating when the appetite is about 80% satisfied.

(*c*) *Chewing:* Regardless of the circumstances, good chewing is one of the most important practices in the way of eating: the more we chew, the better the result.

To maintain a normal, healthy condition, chewing at least 50 times or more for each mouthful is advisable. In the event of sickness, chewing 70–100 times is required. If the sickness is more serious, the amount of chewing should be increased even beyond 100 times per mouthful. Completely mixing the food with saliva is the key to smooth operation of all digestive functions, and this in turn directly serves for the smooth production of healthy blood. In the event that chewing is not possible due to defective teeth or mental weakness, food can be served in mashed form so that it may be mixed slowly with saliva.

(*d*)   *The Process of Change:*   When we follow the above dietary practices according to our condition, it may be difficult to completely and immediately eliminate undesirable foods and drink including complete cessation of the intake of meat, eggs, dairy food, sugar, and other artificial sweets, refined and mass-produced chemicalized foods and beverages. If that is the case, it is recommended to gradually reduce the amount of undesirable food and beverages, and to gradually increase the amount of proper food and beverages. When we have been taking drugs and medicines, it is especially necessary to reduce them gradually, taking a few weeks to several months, depending upon the type of drugs and the extent to which they have been taken. The greater the volume of undesirable food or drugs was, the slower the rate of change should be. However, if we did not have such extreme habits, the previous diet can be changed almost immediately to the new proper diet.

(*e*)   *Control of Recovery Rate:*   There are complementary relationships between the principal food—cereal grains and their products—and all other foods used as supplements—soup, beans, vegetables, seaweed, dessert and beverages. If we wish

---

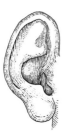

Traditional, balanced ear

The Changing Ear
Modern ears are losing the earlobe; instead, we see ears attached directly to the cheek. The long earlobe has been known as a sign of happiness as well as of balanced physical and mental conditions. The earlobe is developed by proper mineral intake while the absence of an earlobe is due to a lack of minerals and overconsumption of protein. These shapes are formed during embryonic development through the nourishment coming from the placenta. When the mother's nourishment is proper, the baby is born with good earlobes. The upper wing of the ear is developed by more protein, the middle region by more carbohydrate, and the lower region by more minerals.

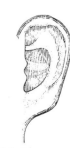

Modern, un-balanced ear

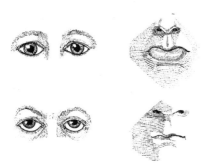

Sanpaku and Swollen Lips
Sanpaku is a term meaning "three whites," indicating the iris is turned upwards, and white can be seen on three sides of the iris. *Sanpaku* on the underside of the iris is traditionally known in oriental countries as an unlucky sign inviting accidents, assassination, and unexpected misfortune. Most people who were assassinated, including Caesar, Hitler, Lincoln, Kennedy, and many others were *sanpaku*, as well as people who were involved in criminal affairs. During babyhood, our eyes were showing three whites on the upper side; during adulthood, our eyes are normal; and at the▶

to accelerate our recovery, generally speaking, we should increase the proportion of principal food and decrease all other side dishes proportionately. On the other hand, if we wish a more gradual recovery, particularly if we have been taking some sort of medication, it is recommended to decrease the amount of principal food and increase all other supplemental foods proportionately.[7] However, the principal food should not be less than 50% of each meal.

B. Transition Period from Previous Habits to a New Dietary Practice

When beginning the practice of proper diet to recover our health, we may experience some physical and mental reactional phenomena during a short transition

---

▶approach of death, everyone becomes *sanpaku*. *Sanpaku* is now very common in modern society —a sign of deterioration of physical and mental conditions.

The condition of the lower lip is directly related to the overall general condition of the intestines. Smoothly functioning intestines are shown by a tight lower lip. When the intestines become enlarged due to improper diet, the lower lip becomes expanded. Especially the over-consumption of yin food such as fruits, potatoes, sugars, fatty and greasy food, and liquid, enlarge both the intestines and the lower lip. Expanded lower lips indicate stagnation and constipation in the intestines. Nine out of ten modern people are suffering from intestinal troubles.

[7] In this sense, not only the macrobiotic way of eating for the recovery of health, but also for any normal daily diet, can be categorized into ten ways of eating, as George Ohsawa described in the accompanying chart (from his book, *Zen Macrobiotics*):

Diet No.	Cereals	Vegetables Sauteed	Soup	Animal	Salads Fruits	Dessert	Beverages
7	100%	—	—	—	—	—	As little as possible, but comfortable
6	90%	10%	—	—	—	—	
5	80%	20%	—	—	—	—	
4	70%	20%	10%	—	—	—	,,
3	60%	30%	10%	—	—	—	,,
2	50%	30%	10%	10%	—	—	,,
1	40%	30%	10%	20%	—	—	,,
−1	30%	30%	10%	20%	10%	—	,,
−2	20%	30%	10%	25%	10%	5%	,,
−3	10%	30%	10%	30%	15%	5%	,,

Is has been the common practice in oriental countries and in ancient societies throughout the world, that the majority of food was cereal grains and their products: brown rice in oriental countries; corn in the American continents; wheat, oats, millet, barley and rye as well as brown rice in European countries; buckwheat in northeastern Europe. Often, these grains and their products were eaten with almost no side dishes for a period of up to ten days, in order to re-orient people's physical and mental conditions. A small volume of seasonings and condiments, and a reasonable volume of beverages, were used as a part of such practices. At that time, these whole cereal grains and their products were prepared in various ways, in the form of gruel, pancakes, bread, noodles, chapati, and other forms. However, the practice of such a diet consisting of 100% whole grains should not continue longer than two weeks unless under experienced supervision. In normal daily life, the principal food can fluctuate between 30% and 70% of each meal, and supplemental food can be adjusted accordingly, depending upon our daily activities and social environment. However, the greater the proportion of principal food, the more balance is achieved among physical, mental, and spiritual capacities.

period, usually lasting from three to ten days, and in some cases up to four months. Such physical and mental reactions have various manifestations, but none of them have any harmful influence upon our life. Usually such reactions are almost negligible, if our native constitution is strong and well-structured, due to our mother's healthy practice of diet and our family's way of life, and especially if the condition of our digestive system has not been affected by any sickness and we have not had unhealthy dietary habits in the past. More pronounced reactions, physical and mental, would generally be experienced by people who have had the following conditions: (1) chaotic dietary habits, especially during the embryonic and childhood periods; (2) intake of many chemicals—not only through modern artificial and chemicalized food, but also as drugs and medications; and (3) those who received surgical operations, especially the removal of parts of organs and glands—such as the tonsils, appendix, ovaries, gall bladder, spleen, and others. In the case of women, an abortion also adversely affects physical and mental strength.

We should not worry if we experience these physical and mental reactional phenomena; they are, in fact, usually desirable, since most of them are either symptomatic manifestations of the recovery process, or the elimination of accumulated toxins from our body. These reactions may be generally classed as follows:

(1) *General fatigue:* A feeling of general fatigue may especially arise among people who have been eating an excessive amount of animal protein and fat. Their previous condition of energetic activity was the result of the vigorous caloric discharge of these excessive foods, rather than a more healthy, balanced, and peaceful way of activity. Often these people initially experience physical tiredness and slight mental depression until the new diet starts to serve as an energy supply for activity. Such a period of fatigue usually ends within a month.

(2) *Pains and Aches:* Pains and aches may be sometimes experienced, especially by people who have been taking excessive liquid, sugar, fruits, or any other extremely yin quality of food and beverages. These pains and aches—such as headaches and pains in the area of the intestines, kidneys, and chest—occur because of the gradual contraction of abnormally expanded tissues and nerve cells. These aches and pains disappear—either gradually or suddenly—as soon as these abnormally expanded areas return to a normal condition, which usually takes between three and fourteen days, depending upon the previous condition.

(3) *Fever, Chills, and Coughing:* As the new health-promoting diet starts to form a more sound quality of blood, previous excessive substances—excessive vol-

---

Renewal of Blood
Human blood is composed of red blood cells, white blood cells, blood platelets, and plasma (the fluid part). When a new type of diet starts to change the quality of the blood, all of these cells change, taking different lengths of time:

Blood plasma—up to approximately 10 days
White blood cells—approximately 20 to 80 days
Red blood cells—approximately 120 days

Accordingly, after a 10-day practice of the new diet, the change of general physical and mental orientation towards a new direction has already begun and it is completed in approximately four months.

ume of liquid, fat, and many other things—begin to be discharged. If at that time the functions of the kidneys, urinary system, and respiratory system have not yet recovered to normal condition, this necessary discharge sometimes takes instead the form of fever, chills, or coughing. These ways of discharge, however, are usually temporary and disappear in several days without any special treatment.

(4) *Abnormal Sweating and Frequent Urination:* As in the symptoms described above, unusual sweating may be experienced by some people from time to time, for a period of several months, and other people may experience unusually frequent urination. In their previous diets, these people have been taking excessive liquid in the form of water, various beverages, alcohol, fruits, fruit juices, milk and other dairy food. By reducing these excessive liquids and fats accumulated in the form of liquid, the body returns to a normal, balanced, healthy condition. These discharges eventually cease; at that time, metabolic balance within various organs and systems has been gradually restored. In the case of chronic diseases, urination is often accompanied by unpleasant odors or unusual colors. For example, in the case of cancer, the urine may be an unusually dark brown.

(5) *Skin Discharge and Unusual Body Odors:* Among the forms of elimination of toxins and fat accumulated in the body is the discharge of unusual odors—usually suggesting rotten and decayed matter—from the entire body surface, through breathing, urination or bowel movements and often, in the case of women, through vaginal discharges. This usually occurs among people who were previously taking excessive volumes of animal fat, dairy food and sugar. In addition, some people experience—for only short periods—skin rashes, reddish swelling at the tips of the fingers and toes, boils, and tumors. These types of eliminations arise especially among people who have taken animal fat, dairy food, sugar, chemicals, spices, and among those who have had chronic malfunctions of the intestines, kidneys, and liver. However, these eliminations naturally heal and usually disappear within a few months without any special attention.

(6) *Diarrhea or Constipation:* People who have had chronically disturbed intestinal conditions due to previous improper dietary habits, may temporarily experience either diarrhea (usually for several days) or constipation (for a period lasting up to 20 days). In this case, diarrhea is a form of discharge of accumulated stagnated matter in the intestines, including unabsorbed food, fat, mucous and liquid. Constipation is the result of a process of contraction of the intestinal tube, which was abnormally expanded due to the previous diet. As this contraction restores normal elasticity to the intestinal tube, the elimination of bowels resumes. No

---

Cause of Baldness

Baldness arises at two different regions on the head. Some cases arise at the peripheral regions of the head, generally starting from the upper region of the forehead—yin ($\triangledown$) area. Other cases arise from the central or top part of the head—yang ($\triangle$) area. The former case is due to the excessive intake of yin food and beverages, including fruits, fruit juices, soft drinks, liquid, and alcohol. The latter case is due to excessive consumption of animal food and salts including meat, eggs, and cheese. In the latter case, strong alcohol often contributes as an additional cause. Even after twenty years of baldness, hair can be restored through the macrobiotic way of eating for a few years.

special treatment is necessary, unless there is a feeling of cloudiness in the head because of the lack of elimination.

(7) *Decrease of Sexual Desire and Vitality:*   There are some people who may feel a weakening of sexual vitality or a decrease of sexual appetite, but not necessarily accompanied by a feeling of fatigue. The reason for such a decline in sexual vitality and desire is that the body functions are working more for the elimination of various sick factors from all parts of the body, and excessive vitality is not available to be used for sexual activity. Also, in some cases, the sexual organs are being actively healed by the new quality of blood, and are not yet prepared to resume normal activity. These conditions, however, last only for a short period, usually a few weeks and, at most, a few months. As soon as this period is over, healthy vitality and desire for sexual activity return.

(8) *Temporary Cessation of Menstruation:*   In some women, there may be a temporary cessation of menstruation. The reason for this cessation is that in the healing process of the entire body, the vital organs, especially those of the respiratory, digestive, excretory and circulatory systems, need to be improved first. Less vital functions, including reproductive activities, are healed later. The period of cessation of menstruation varies, depending upon the individual; a longer time is to be expected for those whose reproductive systems and functions had been in unhealthy conditions, including chronic menstrual irregularity. However, when menstruation begins anew, it is healthy and natural, following the 28-day lunar cycle, and with no discomfort. Mental clarity and emotional calm are enjoyed, as well as physical flexibility.

(9) *Mental Irritability:*   Some people who have been taking drugs and medications for long periods experience emotional irritability after changing their dietary practices. This irritability reflects adjustments taking place in the blood and various body functions, following the change to the different quality of food, and generally passes within one week to several weeks, depending upon how deeply affected the body systems were by the previous habitual use of such drugs and medications. The consumption of sugar, coffee, and alcohol for long periods, as well as long-time smoking, also produce a temporary emotional irritability when the new diet is practiced.

(10) *Other Possible Transitory Experiences:*   In addition to the above conditions, some people may experience other manifestations of adjustment such as: (1) some hair falling out, which naturally restores itself later; (2) fragmental dreams—a sign of discharging past sicknesses, which will stop naturally, resulting in normal deep sleep; (3) a feeling of coldness—especially in the winter season during the first year of the new diet—resulting from the contraction of the surface skin. This will change naturally towards a feeling of warmness in the winter and coolness in the summer, within a few years; and (4) changes in perception and sensitivity may be temporarily experienced, including the sense of touch, taste, smell, hearing, and vision.

All of these above symptoms vary from person to person, depending upon individual constitution and condition, and usually require no special treatment, naturally ceasing as the new order of physical, mental and spiritual function begins to work.

In the event that the symptoms are severe, dietary practice in the new direction can be modified with the continuous consumption of some previous food in small volume—about 10% to 30% of the meal.

During this transition period, there are some people who crave the tastes, textures, odors and other characteristics of their previous food and drink. If such cravings disturb one emotionally, they would accordingly hinder the normal mental and physical activities. If such cravings cannot be comfortably satisfied within the dimensions of the new diet, it is necessary to take some of the previous type of food from time to time until such cravings eventually disappear. Often during this period a person may suffer from guilt feelings as if he or she is committing a sin by taking the previous types of wrong food and drink. This guilty conscience should be forgotten and a more relaxed attitude must be taken since some of the previous types of food may be needed until the new diet becomes well-established as a foundation for physical, mental, and spiritual activities. However, it is generally far better for the improvement of health to satisfy such cravings by replacing previous wrong quality of food and drink with a better quality. The following listing may serve as a guide in substituting better-quality foods for those wrong foods we crave:

Cravings	Replacement	Goal
Sugar, honey, chocolate, and other sweeteners	Rice honey, barley malt, maple syrup, carob	Natural sweetening from whole cereal grains and vegetables
Meat, such as beef and pork; eggs	Organic poultry, especially the white meat of birds; organic eggs	Fish and seafood, especially white meat
Dairy food, cheese, milk, cream, butter	Organic dairy food, in small volume; nuts, nut butters	Organic and traditional soybean products such as *miso*, *tofu*, soy milk, and other bean products; sesame butter and other seed butters
Tropical and semitropical fruits and artificial fruit juices	Organic fruits and fruit juices	Organic fruits and fruit juices in small volume, and limited to only locally and seasonally grown
Alcoholic beverages including liquor, wines, and beers	Traditionally brewed alcoholic beverages, especially brewed from organic cereal grains, such as beer and *sake*	Mild alcoholic beverages brewed from organic cereal grains, used only in small volume from time to time
Coffee, aromatic stimulant beverages and soft drinks	Herb teas of less aromatic and stimulant effects	*Bancha* twig tea, *Mu* tea and other herb teas of non-aromatic stimulant effects

C. Medicinal Use of Common Food

In addition to the adjustment of atmospheric conditions, physical and mental activities, and change of climate, as well as dietary practices, there may sometimes be a need for some traditional natural applications to hasten improvement. These methods can be called home medicine or folk treatment. All of them have been developed through the actual experiences of people for many centuries. They are simple and practical enough for anyone to use in usual living circumstances. They are also sufficiently useful and effective so that often people do not need constant medical attention.

All materials used for such treatments are, in most cases, common daily food items and usual household supplies, easily obtainable at any time. All traditional races and cultures have relied upon such natural ways of healing, and some of these methods are often more effective than modern medicine, without producing any side effects. They are also much more economical than the modern way of treatment. Some examples of such medicinal uses of common foods that have been used traditionally for many centuries in Far Eastern countries are as follows:

(1) *Ginger Fomentation (Ginger Compress)*—to stimulate blood and body fluid circulation and to dissolve stagnation.

> Grate fresh ginger and place in a cheesecloth sack. Squeeze out ginger liquid in hot water (kept just below the boiling point). Dip towel into ginger water, wring out tightly, and apply—hot—directly to the necessary area. Every 2–3 minutes, change to fresh hot towel until the skin becomes red.

(2) *Mustard Plaster*—to stimulate blood and body fluid circulation and to release stagnation.

> Add hot water to dry mustard and stir well. Spread this mixture on a paper towel, and sandwich the paper towel between two bath towels (thick cotton towels). Apply "sandwich" to the skin. After skin becomes warm and red, remove application.

(3) *Tofu Plaster*—more effective than an ice pack to draw out fever.

> Squeeze out water from *tofu*; mash *tofu* and add 10%–20% pastry flour and 5% grated ginger. Mix all ingredients very well. Apply directly to body. Change every 2–3 hours.

(4) *Taro Potato Plaster (Albi Plaster) or Common Potato and Vegetable Plaster* — to draw out pus and stagnant blood from tumors, boils, and the like.

> Remove hairy skin from the taro potato and grate the white interior. Mix with 5% grated fresh ginger. Spread mixture 1/2 inch thick on a piece of cotton linen, and apply the potato side directly to the tumor or skin. Change every 4 hours. Before and after this application, a ginger fomentation may be used to warm up the body. In the event taro potato (albi) is not available, grated fresh potato 50% and mashed green leafy vegetables 50%, mixed thoroughly, can be applied as a substitute. If the mixture does not hold together well to make a paste, mix in 10–20% white flour until sticky.

(5) *Lotus Root Plaster*—to drain stagnated mucus from the sinuses, nose, throat and bronchi.

> Grate fresh lotus root and mix with 10%–15% pastry flour and 5% grated fresh ginger. Spread 1/2 inch thick on cotton linen. Apply lotus root side directly to the chosen place. Keep on for several hours or overnight. Repeat daily for several days.

(6) *Buckwheat Plaster*—to eliminate retained water and other fluid.

> Mix buckwheat flour with sesame oil and hot water to form a stiff hard dough. Apply, 1/2 inch thick, directly to swollen place. When it draws out fluid, the

dough becomes soft and watery. Then replace with a new, stiff dough. Change every 3–4 hours.

(7) *Carp Plaster*—to reduce high fever such as in pneumonia.

Crush and mash the head and body of a live carp. Mix with a small volume of white wheat flour. Spread this mixture on oiled paper and apply to the chest. In the case of pneumonia, drink 1 to 2 teaspoons of the carp's blood, and then apply the plaster. After the carp plaster is made, measure the body temperature every half hour until it reaches normal. At that time, immediately remove the carp plaster.

(8) *Salt Pack*—to heat any part of the body; for example, the abdominal area in case of diarrhea.

Roast salt in a dry pan until hot. Wrap heated salt in a thick cotton linen or a towel. Apply to the necessary area. Change when it starts to cool.

(9) *Daikon* (*Long White Radish*) *Drink No. 1*—to reduce fever by inducing sweating.

Mix half a cup of grated fresh *daikon* with 1 tablespoon *tamari* soy sauce and 1/4 teaspoon grated ginger. Pour hot *bancha* tea over this mixture to cover, and stir well. Drink while hot.

Daikon (*Long White Radish*) *Drink No. 2*—to prompt urination.
Grate *daikon* and squeeze out the juice using a piece of cheesecloth. Mix 2 tablespoons of this juice with 6 tablespoons of hot water. Add a pinch of sea salt. Boil all ingredients together, then drink. (Never use without boiling.) Take only once a day, and do not use more than three times without proper supervision.

(10) *Ranshio*—to strengthen the heart, stimulate heart beat and blood circulation.

Break a raw egg and mix very well with one tablespoon *tamari* soy sauce.
Drink slowly. (Use only once a day and do not use more than three days.)

(11) *Tamari Bancha Tea*—to strengthen the blood if it is in an acidic condition, and to prompt blood circulation; to relieve fatigue.

Pour 1 cup hot *bancha* twig tea over 1–2 teaspoons of *tamari* soy sauce. Stir well and drink while hot.

(12) *Salt Bancha Tea*—to loosen stagnation in the nasal cavity and to cleanse the vaginal region.

Put enough sea salt in warm *bancha* tea (body temperature) to make it a little less salty than sea water. Use this liquid to wash deep inside the nasal cavity through the nostrils, or use for douching in the vaginal region. This salt *bancha* tea can be used also for washing troubled eyes.

(13) *Ume-Sho-Bancha*—to strengthen the blood and the circulation through the regulation of digestion.

Pour 1 cup *bancha* tea over the meat of 1/2 to 1 *umeboshi* plum and 1 teaspoon *tamari* soy sauce. Stir well and drink while hot.

(14) *Kuzu* (*Kudzu*) *Drink*—to strengthen digestion and vitality, and to relieve general fatigue.

Bring to a boil one cup of water in which 1 heaping teaspoon of *kuzu* root powder has been dissolved. Simmer, stir constantly, until it becomes a transparent gelatin, and then stir in 1 teaspoon *tamari* soy sauce. Drink while hot.

(15) *Ume-Sho-Kuzu (Kudzu) Drink*—to strengthen digestion and revitalize energy; also, to regulate the intestinal condition.

Prepare *Kuzu* Drink as above, adding the meat of 1/2 to 1 *umeboshi* plum along with the soy sauce. 1/8 teaspoon grated fresh ginger may also be added.

(16) *Umeboshi Plum, or Baked Umeboshi Plum, or Powder of Baked Umeboshi Plum Pit*—to neutralize overacidity and relieve intestinal problems, including those caused by microorganisms.

Take 2–3 *umeboshi* plums with *bancha* twig tea; or, bake *umeboshi* plums or their pits in the oven until they become completely black. In the case of pits, crush them into powder and take 1 tablespoon with a little hot water or tea.

(17) *Denshi (Dentie)*—to prevent any tooth trouble, and to stop any bleeding by inducing contraction of expanded blood capillaries.

Bake an eggplant, particularly the cap portion, until it becomes completely black. Crush into powder and mix well with 30%–50% roasted sea salt. Use daily as tooth powder or apply to any bleeding area—even inside the nostrils in the case of nosebleed (by inserting wet tissue dipped in *dentie* into nostril).

(18) *Gomashio (Sesame Salt)*—to strengthen digestion and intestinal absorption as well as blood quality, and to relieve general fatigue and pains such as headache and toothache.

For a home remedy, mix 3 to 4 parts roasted sesame seeds with 1 part roasted sea salt. (For daily use at meals as a condiment, use 8–14 parts sesame seeds to 1 part sea salt.) Grind in a *suribachi* (mortar and pestle) slowly and evenly, crushing all seeds well but not completely to powder form. Take one teaspoon of *gomashio* once or twice a day for several days. This may be taken together with hot *bancha* twig tea or with hot water, or sprinkled over cereal grains in the course of the meal.

(19) *Sesame Oil*—to induce elimination of stagnated bowels and to draw out retained water.

In order to induce the discharge of stagnated bowels, take 1–2 tablespoons of raw sesame oil on an empty stomach. In order to eliminate water retention in the eyes, put a drop or two of pure sesame oil in the eyes with an eyedropper, preferably before sleeping. Continue several days to a few weeks until eyes improve. For this use, pure sesame oil should be boiled and strained with sanitized cheesecloth to remove any impurities.

(20) *Ginger Sesame Oil*—to activate the functioning of the blood capillaries, circulation, and nervous reactions; and to relieve aches and pains.

Mix grated fresh ginger with an equal amount of sesame oil. Dip cotton linen into this ginger sesame oil and strongly rub the necessary area of the skin.

(21) *Raw Brown Rice and Seeds*—to eliminate various worms.

Skip breakfast and lunch. On an empty stomach, take a handful of raw brown rice with half a handful of raw seeds such as pumpkin seeds or sunflower seeds, and another half-handful of chopped raw onion, scallion, or garlic. Chew everything well and swallow. Repeat for 2–3 days.

(22) *Brown Rice Cream*—to supply nourishment and energy when exhausted and when there is no digestive ability.

Roast brown rice evenly until all grains become a yellowish color. To one part rice, add a very small amount of sea salt and 3–6 parts water, and pressure cook at least two hours. Place cooked soft brown rice gruel in sanitized cheesecloth and squeeze out the creamy part of the rice. Eat with a small volume of condiment, such as *umeboshi* plum, *gomashio* (sesame salt), *tekka*, or kelp or other seaweed powder.

(23) *Grated Daikon (Long White Radish)*[8]—to aid digestion, especially of fatty, oily, heavy food, animal food and other foods.

Grate fresh *daikon* (if not available, use red radish or turnip) and eat about 1 tablespoon with several drops of *tamari* soy sauce.

(24) *Dried Daikon Leaves*—to warm the body temperature; especially helpful for women's skin and sexual metabolism. It also aids in extracting body odors and excessive oils, and in clearing up various skin diseases caused by animal food.

Dry some fresh *daikon* leaves in the house, away from sunlight, until they become brown and brittle. (If *daikon* leaves are not available, turnip greens may be used instead.) Boil 4–5 bunches of leaves with about 4–5 quarts of water until the water turns brown. Add a handful of sea salt and stir well, and use in one of the following ways:

1. Dip cotton linen into this hot liquid and lightly squeeze. Apply on affected area of skin. Make repeated applications until skin becomes completely red.

2. Pour this hot liquid into a hot bath. Mix well; immerse body in this water.

3. To treat troubles of women's sexual organs, sit in the bathtub with the bath as described above, only up to the waist, for about 10 minutes until the whole body becomes warm and starts to sweat, covering the upper part of the body with a towel. Repeat several days up to 10 days as needed.

4. This liquid can be strained and used as a douche to eliminate mucus and fat accumulated in the regions of the uterus and vagina.

(25) *Salt Water*—(1) cold salt water may be used to contract the skin surface, especially in the case of burns; (2) warm salt water may be used to clean the rectum, colon and vagina.

1. When the skin is damaged by fire, immediately soak the burned area in cold salt water until irritation completely disappears; then apply vegetable oil on the affected area to seal from the air.

2. For constipation or mucus and fat accumulations in the rectum, colon, and vaginal regions, use warm salt water (body temperature) as an enema or douche.

(26) *Juice of Scallion, Onion, or Daikon*—to neutralize toxins caused by bee

---

[8] *Traditional Uses of Grated Daikon:* In oriental countries, it has been the custom for many centuries to serve grated fresh *daikon* or shredded fresh *daikon* along with a dish of *tempura* (deep-fried vegetables or seafood), *sashimi* (sliced fresh raw fish), *mochi* (pounded sweet rice cakes) and other heavy food.

stings and insect bites.

Cut scallion, onion, or *daikon*, or their greens, and squeeze out the juice. (If those vegetables are not available, red radish may be used.) Rub juice strongly on the affected area.

4. Mental Disorders: Cause and Approach

A. *Relation between Body and Mind*

In the modern world, mental problems are approached as though they were independent from physical problems. However, as we see in traditional medicine, particularly in the Orient, the approach to mental problems is not separate from the approach to physical problems. Physical sicknesses are immediate causes of mental disturbances, and mental troubles immediately affect the physical condition. Both mental and physical problems are two different manifestations arising from the same root: a disorderly way of life, including the habitual practice of improper diet, and a lack of balance in mental and physical activities.

In oriental medicine, it has been traditionally known that each major organ and its sickness is connected to each major mental phenomenon. These physical and mental phenomena have been understood as progressive interrelated developments, taking place according to the five transformation stages of interaction between yin (centrifugal) and yang (centripetal) tendencies:

(1) Unhealthy conditions of the liver and gall bladder produce short temper and anger, while their healthy conditions produce patience and endurance.

(2) Unhealthy conditions of the heart and small intestines produce excitement and excessive laughter, while their healthy conditions produce tranquility and gentleness.

(3) Unhealthy conditions of the spleen, pancreas and stomach produce emotional irritability and conceptual skepticism, while their healthy conditions produce sympathy and understanding.

(4) Unhealthy conditions of the lungs and large intestine produce a feeling of sadness and worry, while their healthy conditions produce a feeling of happiness and security.

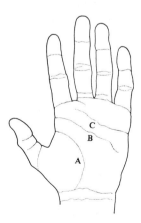

Indications from Lines on the Palm

Line A is showing the digestive and respiratory system; called the *Life Line*.

Line B represents the nervous system; called the *Line of Intellect*.

Line C indicates the circulatory and excretory systems; called the *Line of Emotion*.

All lines should be clear and powerful, if we are in healthy condition. Line A is longest, and Line B is shortest: Line C is in between. These three basic lines as well as many other lines indicate physical, mental, and spiritual constitutions and conditions. The left hand represents the heritage from the father, while the right hand indicates the heritage from the mother.

(5)   Unhealthy conditions of the kidneys and bladder produce fear and depression, while their healthy conditions produce confidence and courage.

The functions of these major organs are also closely related to our various spiritual natures and activities:

(1)   Healthy liver and gall bladder conditions insure spiritual strength and endless pursuit of development.

(2)   A healthy heart and small intestine insure intuitive comprehension and the feeling of oneness.

(3)   Healthy spleen, pancreas, and stomach conditions insure spiritual wisdom and understanding.

(4)   Healthy lungs and large intestines insure spiritual love and unlimited sympathy.

(5)   Healthy kidneys and bladder insure inspiration and a spirit of aspiration.

Fig. 32   Five Stages of Physical and Mental Transformation

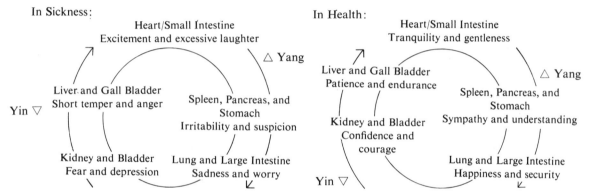

Often, we are conscious of the kinds of dreams we see in the night, and we remember them after we awake. Our food and other physical conditions are also producing such dreams and if our food and other factors are changed, our dreams also change.

Dreams can generally be classified into five different categories:

(1)   *Nightmares:*   Dreams of violence, murder, suffering, bloody scenes; often, the appearance of monsters. Such dreams result from the intake of large amounts of animal food, especially beef, pork, and other mammals' meat. The liver and gall bladder, heart and small intestine are in this case affected to some degree by the heavy intake of animal food.

(2)   *Dreams of Human Events:*   Meeting with people, social events, parties, ceremonies and festivities, arguments and quarrels, and other human affairs. These dreams are resulting from the intake of large amounts of fat and oils which may come from both animal and vegetable sources. In this case, the kidneys, bladder, spleen, pancreas and stomach are more affected.

(3)   *Dreams of Excitement and Destruction:*   Fire, earthquakes, war, and many other kinds of natural and social excitement. These dreams result from the intake of large amounts of hot spices, aromatic stimulant seasonings and beverages, includ-

ing alcohol; also, excessive intake of baked and burned food. In this case the liver, gall bladder, spleen, pancreas, and stomach are more affected.

(4) *Fragmental Dreams:* Floating, misty, disconnected dreams which are easily forgotten, and which make us tired when we awake. These dreams result from the intake of excessive amounts of sugar and other sweets, weak alcohol, excessive volume of liquid, fruit, fruit juices, and often, drugs and medications. In this case, the lungs, large intestines, kidneys and bladder are more affected.

(5) *Dreams of Natural Scenes:* Natural scenery—celestial phenomena such as the sun, moon and stars, wind, rain, snow, mountains, forests, rivers and oceans. These dreams result from the intake of beans and vegetables, excessively unbalanced in proportion to the principal food—cereal grains; and also from excessive salad, fruits and liquid. In this case, the lungs, large intestine, heart and small intestine are more affected.

Also, dreams such as falling from high places are often caused by excessive eating of tree fruits; dreams of drowning are often caused by excessive intake of liquid before sleeping; and dreams of sexual indulgence are often caused by the intake of excessive amounts of protein and fat.

When we see dreams in the night, we are seeing our surroundings and interpreting them into our impressions by the same brain and nervous functions that are taking place while we are awake. If our brains and nervous functions are disordered, our dreams will also be disordered. In order to see without our personal disordered view, and to interpret our surroundings properly, we must eliminate the causes of our night dreams. The cause of our night dreams is the same as the cause of our day dreams—very simply, an improper way of eating according to an improper way of life.

B. Progressive Development of Mental Disorders

When our dietary practice and our general way of life are not in accord with the change of natural conditions, we begin to develop mental disorders as our physical orientation becomes disordered. These mental disorders can develop gradually in seven progressive stages, as such disordered ways of life continue:

	Yin Cause ($\triangledown$)	*Yang Cause* ($\triangle$)
	Overconsumption of sugar and other sweeteners, fruits, fruit juice, chemicals, most medications, drugs, alcohol, hot spices, dairy food, some vegetables of tropical and semi-tropical origin, excessive liquid.	Overconsumption of meat and other animal food, salt, baked and burned food, insufficient liquid intake.
1st Stage:	General mental fatigue, manifesting in complaining and gradual loss of clear thinking and behavior.	General mental fatigue, manifesting in frequent changing of the mind and gradual loss of steadiness in mind and attitude.

	Yin Cause ($\bigtriangledown$)	*Yang Cause* ($\bigtriangleup$)
2nd Stage:	Feeling of melancholy, gradual loss of ambition and self-confidence; the beginning of forgetfulness and vague memory.	Beginning of rigidity, gradually developing into stubbornness and insistent attention to trivial matters.
3rd Stage:	Emotional irritability and fear, prevailing depression; defensive attitude.	Excitability, short-temper, prevailing discontentment, offensive attitude.
4th Stage:	Suspicion and skepticism, misconceptions and misinterpretation, general retreating attitude.	Conceptualization, producing various "-isms," manifesting delusions in various beliefs.
5th Stage:	Discrimination and prejudice based upon inferiority complex.	Discrimination and prejudice based upon superiority complex.
6th Stage:	Loss of self-discipline; chaos in thinking and attitude; schizophrenic symptoms.	Exclusive indoctrination; egocentric thinking and attitude; paranoid symptoms.
7th Stage:	Yin ($\bigtriangledown$) arrogance: total inability to adapt to the environment; encasing himself in his delusional cage.	Yang ($\bigtriangleup$) arrogance: total inability to accept others—forcing self-justified control on others.

In modern society, the overwhelming majority of people are described in one of the above categories of mental disorders. Modern society is a huge mental clinic, with hundreds of millions of people who are mentally disordered. Political, legal, economic systems and many other social systems in modern society are either (1) accelerating the development of people's mental disorders or (2) regulating people who have chaotic attitudes arising from their mental disorders. Most of modern education is especially serving both functions, alienating us from the natural order of our environment, from the memory of our origin in this universe, and even from each other in this human society.

For the recovery of humanity from present-day disorders—physical, mental, and spiritual—we need a total approach through our own deep self-reflection upon our way of life, including our dietary practice and orientation of our civilization as a whole. Otherwise, personal health may be achieved, but mankind as a whole will continue to suffer and eventually cease to exist through biological and social extinction.

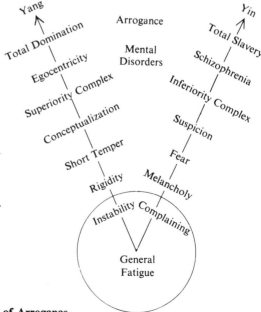

Fig. 33 The Development of Arrogance

Progressive Development Toward Cancer

Modern society is suffering with constantly increasing cases of various cancers. The prevalence of cancer is reaching an epidemic level, and it is estimated that in the United States, one out of every four persons will suffer from cancer during his or her lifetime. Many efforts have been devoted to discovering the cause and method of the effective healing of this universal sickness. Many theories and assumptions have been presented on the cause of cancer—the virus theory, the mutation theory, the hereditary theory, the stimulus theory, the chemical and radiation theories, and others. However, the cause of cancer is nothing more than modern dietary habits leading to an inadequate quality of blood and body fluid, which result in the production of abnormal cells. The origin of cancer is the modern way of living in general, which has everywhere become artificial and removed from the natural environment.

Though cancer symptoms are yin because of the rapid increase and differentiation of cancer cells, the cause of cancer may be either (1) excessive consumption of yin food and beverages, (2) excessive consumption of yang food and beverages, or (3) excessive consumption of both extremes. The first case, yin dietary cause, is, practically speaking, excessive intake for a long duration of chemicalized food and drinks, sugar, chocolate, honey, and artificial sweeteners, soft drinks, milk and other dairy food, including butter, oil and fat of both animal and vegetable origins, refined white grains and flour products, hot spices, stimulant and aromatic beverages, wine and other alcoholic beverages, and excessive intake of tropical and semi-tropical fruits and fruit juices, as well as such vegetables of tropical origin as tomatoes and potatoes.

The yang dietary cause of cancer is the excessive consumption of meat, eggs, and some cheese, as well as the overconsumption of salt, especially used with animal food.

Cancer caused by both yin and yang extremes in dietary habits means the continuous overconsumption of foods of both of the above categories.

Generally, cancer created by a yin cause is produced in the more yin, expanded and soft parts of the body—the skin, esophagus, breast, stomach wall, intestinal vessels, especially the ascending and transverse colon, and the bladder.

Cancer produced by yang causes generally appears in more yang, compacted and hard parts of the body—the liver, duodenum, pancreas, kidneys, and brain.

Cancer caused by extremes of both yin and yang generally appears in other areas—for example, the throat, lungs, uterus, prostate, descending colon, and rectum.

However, in the case of leukemia (blood cancer), the main cause is excessive consumption of yin types of foods; and lymphatic cancer is caused by both extremes.

Of course, all cancers have both extremes to some extent, and for this very reason it is very difficult to heal cancer by any specific type of treatment or medication.

Cancer never arises suddenly but develops progressively over a long period. There are many people in modern society who are going in the direction of cancer, with or without their own knowledge. Cancer develops progressively according to the following stages:

1st Stage—Normal Health: Under normal circumstances, we maintain a balance in our blood of minerals, protein, fat, carbohydrates, vitamins, enzymes and other factors, as well as maintaining the balance between acidity and alkalinity, through our food and our buffer actions. Normal physical activities also serve to keep this balance. Any excessive consumption which tends to create toxic effects is discharged through breathing, urination, sweating, and other activities.

2nd Stage—Abnormal Discharge: If we continue to consume excessive amounts of unsuitable food or beverages, the toxins produced are eliminated through additional functions of discharge, producing abnormal symptoms such as skin disease, excessive sweating, coughing, and fever. In this stage, various sicknesses of adjustment arise.

3rd Stage—Accumulation and Storage: When we further continue to take excessively disordered food and beverages, we start to accumulate these excesses within our body in the form of mucus, fat, and protein. These accumulations first gather in areas and passages directly connected to the external environment. Mucus accumulates in the sinus and nasal cavities and ears; fat accumulates in the breasts; mucus and fat gather in the lungs and bronchi; mucus and fat gather in the ovaries, uterus, and vaginal region; and also mucus and fat accumulate in the kidneys, urinary tubes, and bladder. These accumulations cause headache, running nose, hay fever, hearing difficulties, breathing difficulties, hardening of the breast, water retention, vaginal discharge, and many other symptoms.

4th Stage—Formation of Cysts, Stones, and Tumors: When stored excess cannot be discharged, it becomes stagnant, and gradually forms cysts, stones, and tumors. Breast cysts, kidney and gall stones, mucus calcification in the sinuses, and various tumors arise in this stage. Especially extreme yin food which lowers body temperature, such as fruit juice, soft drinks, icy cold beverages, and ice cream, accelerates calcification and stone formation.

5th Stage—The Creation of Cancer: If the habitual intake of any excess is continued beyond the previous stage, the concentration of the excess in one location of the body starts to take place. This localization is made to allow all other parts of the body to continue functioning properly. Because of the body's increasing inability to balance its condition through normal discharge, unhealthy blood cells gather and form a mass of cancer cells. Continuation of improper food further causes the mass to enlarge or the cancerous cells to spread.

The speed of this progressive development is faster among people who have received operations in the past such as the removal of the tonsils, adenoids, appendix, one or both kidneys, gall bladder, spleen, and also operation for abortion. These prolonged uses of medicine and these operations have caused an inability of the body to prevent the progressive development towards cancer. The 2nd, 3rd, and 4th stages described above may be considered as pre-cancerous conditions. Although cancer may be removed by operation, destroyed by radiation therapy, or controlled by chemotherapy, if the cause of cancer —wrong dietary practice—is not corrected, cancer may arise again at any place in the body.

For the prevention and healing of cancer, we must undertake a drastic improvement of our dietary habits with self-reflection upon our present way of life. The macrobiotic way of life, including its dietary practice, is the most certain way to approach cancer.

Spectroscopic Classification of Elements in a Logarithmic Spiral

1. The above spirallic arrangement of major elements is made according to spectroscopic examination of color waves. Approximately 8,000 Å to 5,000 Å is the area of yang elements, and approximately, 5,000 Å to 3,500 Å for yin elements. According to this chart, elements occupying the positions in opposite orbits can combine easily due to the principle of attraction between yin and yang; and elements occupying a similar position have difficulty combining with each other unless technical changes of temperature, pressure, or nature are applied.

2. Elements occupying peripheral areas are more yin and lighter, while elements located at more central areas are more yang and heavier. Elements belonging in the most central orbits are radioactive, tending to return to the outer orbits, in the same way the sun is radiating its energy outwards in the solar system. Most balanced elements are found in the fourth orbit, and some of them are magnetic, such as iron (Fe), cobalt (Co), and nickel (Ni).

3. This spirallic chart reveals that lighter elements are gradually transmuting towards heavier elements and heavier elements are in turn transmuting back into lighter elements, though it may take some thousands to millions of years in its natural process. Especially, the transmuting speed of peripheral elements is much slower than that of central elements.

4. The precise chart of classification of the elements by yin and yang should be considered together with this spectroscopic examination, including other factors such as the nature of chemical reactions, and freezing, melting, and boiling temperatures. Knowing the yin and yang natures of elements, we are able to reveal all laws and phenomena—chemical and biochemical, geological and biological—as well as the order of change.

chapter 6

One Peaceful World

> When an individual person masters himself,
> his family becomes happy.
> When the family is happy, society becomes
> healthy.
> When society is healthy, the world becomes
> peaceful.
>
> January, 1977

1. The Biological Revolution of Humanity

We modern men and women are all facing a biological crisis. The most critical problem confronting us today is not political, economic, religious, or ideological; it is the question of whether the human race can continue to survive and develop, or whether it will rapidly degenerate and eventually become extinct. A biological Flood of Noah is prevailing everywhere throughout the so-called modern civilized society. Village to village, town to town, country to country, all people are suffering physical, mental, and spiritual disorders. A world-wide current of biological degeneration is involving everyone, everywhere.

No one who lives within modern civilization is exempt from this world-wide degeneration. From a street beggar to a millionaire, from the newborn to the aged, housewives to businessmen, workers to national leaders—whether black or white, oriental or occidental, Christian or Buddhist, capitalist or socialist, rich or poor, man or woman—everyone is on trial at this critical time. Governmental policies, religious teachings, educational programs, social systems, all seem ineffective in meeting this universal crisis.

If we wish to continue our existence on this earth, it is necessary to devote our best possible efforts toward the reconstruction of humanity on all levels—individual, family, community, national, and international. When a course of degeneration is turned instead in the direction of the continuous existence and future development of mankind through these efforts, a new world will begin, based on a sound biological foundation with new social, ideological, and spiritual orientations. Otherwise, there shall be no peace in the world; there shall be no hope for the future of mankind.

A. Reorientation of the Individual
In order to recover and develop our health, physically, mentally, and spiritually, every person should re-orient his way of life:

(1) We should reflect upon our own daily life, whether we are pursuing only sensory pleasure and emotional comfort, forgetting our native potential for greater happiness and higher freedom.

(2)   We should reflect further upon our daily food and drink, as to whether they are really proper to produce the best quality of blood and cells as well as to secure our best mental and spiritual conditions.

(3)   We should further reflect upon our thought and behavior, towards our parents, family, friends, and other people as to whether our respect and love are really dedicated from our heart, and whether our behavior towards them is really serving for their health and happiness.

(4)   We should also reflect upon our direction, as to whether or not we are constructing societies and civilizations against the order of nature, ignoring the conditions of the environment.

(5)   We should reflect, finally, upon our understanding: do we know where we have come from and where we are going in this infinite universe?

We should recover our native and intuitive memory and understanding of the infinite order of the universe, its mechanism of change, and its manifestation in our human life and daily activities. The beginning of self-recovery from all personal unhappiness including physical and mental disorders, is our understanding of the perpetual order of yin and yang, their dialectic and dynamic change governing every phenomenon.

In order to release ourselves from all physical and mental sicknesses, changing our degenerative tendencies towards health and happiness, we must first apply our understanding of yin and yang to our daily dietary practice—how to choose, prepare, and take our food and drink. Because of this proper practice, our blood and body become of sound condition, and this develops our mental and spiritual well-being with the following favorable results:

(1)   Without any other preventative measures, we are able to maintain our physical health, suffering no serious sickness.

(2)   Without any other special mental-psychological training, we are able to establish a sound mentality, experiencing no delusions and other mental disorders.

(3)   Without any other special efforts, we are able to understand with ease any subject which we desire to learn.

(4)   Without any special education, we are naturally able to develop a spirit of love for other people and of harmony with our environment.

(5)   Without imposing upon ourselves any special restriction, we do not harbor any thoughts of destruction and violence.

(6)   Without any special experience, we are naturally inspired with the spirit of ambition and endless aspiration, enduring any hardship with gratitude.

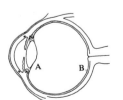

Cause of Myopia

Myopia (nearsightedness) results from two causes: (1) swelling of the lense (A) due to vertical contraction ($\triangle$), and (2) expansion of the eyeball ($\triangledown$) which draws back the position of the retina (B). In both cases the image of the object viewed focuses not on the retina but in front of the retina. These symptoms are called nearsightedness. The former case is due to excessive intake of yang food such as animal food and salts, and the latter case is caused by the excessive intake of yin food and beverages such as sugar, fruits, fruit juices, soft drinks, liquid, drugs, and chemicals.

(7)   Without any other training, we are able to experience our oneness with every being and all phenomena surrounding us.

Food is creating us. If food is proper, we are naturally more energetic physically, comfortable emotionally, and elevated spiritually. If food is not proper, our health declines, emotions are disturbed and our spirit becomes chaotic. Personal feelings, social relations, and our approach to any problems are influenced by what we eat. When we feel any frustration and disturbance, when we meet any difficulty and hardship, we should first reflect upon what we have been eating. Our physical and mental habits as well as tendencies in our thinking and capacities of our consciousness all depend upon what we have been eating for a long period, up to the present. To change our food is to wholly change ourselves. By doing so, we orient our destiny.

In the way of personal eating, there are three stages:

(1)   *Eating to recover from physical and mental disorders*

In this case the way of eating including the selection, preparation, and manner of eating of our food should be strictly disciplined according to the required adjustments, along with the understanding of balance, yin and yang, to reach the state of greatest harmony with the environment.

(2)   *Eating to maintain health and energetic activities, physically and mentally*

In this case, our food should be wider in variety and manner of preparation. It may fluctuate within a reasonable scope of balance depending upon activities and social requirements, yet our principal food—whole cereal grains and their products—should be taken every day with the various supplements as side dishes.

(3)   *Eating to develop and realize our dream*

In this case, we adjust freely the kinds, volume, preparation, and time of eating of our foods, according to our dream which we wish to realize. Each food and each way of preparation has certain physical and mental effects. Knowing these characteristics, we freely manage our daily eating to produce our best condition, to continue to see our dream, and to realize it. This way of eating is truly making use of our freedom, and is the highest art with which we can liberate ourselves in all domains.

While we are physically and emotionally in disorder, we are unable to enjoy our

---

Recommendations of Eating According to Dream

To be religious and spiritual—eat vegetable quality of food including whole cereal grains, beans, vegetables, and fruits with the minimum possible amount of animal food.

To be social and businesslike—eat mostly vegetable quality grains and beans, cooked in a standard way, in a wider variety of methods with the addition of a small volume of animal food.

To be suitable for heavy physical labor, eat more volume of food—whole cereal grains, beans, vegetables, and animal food, richly cooked, with a larger volume of liquid.

To be more intellectual—eat whole grains, beans, and vegetables with the occasional addition of a small volume of animal food and fruits.

To be more sensitive and aesthetic—eat mostly vegetable food, including raw salad. Fruits may be added, as well as a little more liquid, and a small volume of animal food if desired.

To be physically active—eat regularly.

To be mentally active—eat less volume.

To be warlike and violent—eat more animal food and sugar, with a variety of food prepared in a disorderly fashion.

life on this earth. We should recover our health as soon as possible and we should begin to pursue our dream with many other people who are also healthy. Life is nothing but endlessly realizing our dream, and if we are not doing so we are seriously ill.

B.   Reorientation of Family and Community

Among all undesirable thoughts and conduct disturbing the family and the community, sickness—physical and mental—is the greatest sin, and health and well-being the greatest liberation. When one person becomes sick, the whole family suffers; and when one family suffers, the whole community becomes unstable. A family which has a sick person has been disoriented for some time. A community which has many sick people has been disordered for a long period.

Sicknesses—physical and mental—never arise without cause: one's own disorderly way of life. Sicknesses are the warning from our intuition (you may say, the voice of God) telling us how wrong our way of life has been. A person suffering from sickness should make reflection, extending his deep apologies to himself, his family, his community and the universe itself. Sentimental consolations, including the presentation of flowers, fruits or candies to a sick person, are not helpful at all. He needs deep concern and warm care to guide him towards the proper understand-

---

Degenerating Modern People

Modern people, because of their excessive intake of liquid, fat, and sugar, as well as animal food and artificially synthesized food, manifest various unbalanced conditions:

(1) Deep horizontal ridges on the forehead (bladder and kidney troubles from excessive liquid, and intestinal weakening from excessive fat);

(2) Vertical ridges between the eyebrows (liver troubles from excessive amounts of food, especially fats);

(3) Raised and shortened eyebrows (tight nervous system and shorter digestive vessels from excessive animal food);

(4) *Sanpaku* eyes (enlargement of eyeballs and expansion of brain nerve cells by excessive liquid, sweets, fruits and soft drinks);

(5) Large eye bags (kidney disorders from excessive liquid and fat);

(6) Enlarged nose (heart disorder from excessive liquid, sugar, animal fat intake);

(7) Extremely large mouth (weak constitution and dilation of digestive vessels by excessive liquid, fruits, and chemicals);

(8) Fattening of face and neck (degeneration of general functions due to excessive animal food and liquid);

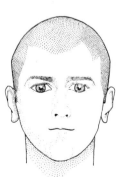

(9) Loss of hair (general physical and mental disorders due to either excessive fruits and liquid or excessive animal food);

(10) Formation of tumors on the head (excessive protein and fat);

(11) Small, pointed ears (small capacity of personality and weak kidneys due to excessive animal food and lack of minerals).

Modern people are now becoming devils, and modern societies are becoming hell; but devils were once angels when they were eating proper food. Lost paradise can be regained through the proper way of life including the proper dietary practice.

ing of why he has to suffer, and to inspire him toward the proper food and nourishment as a basis for the way of life which he should follow hereafter.

Beyond anything else, the orientation of family and community should be directed towards maintaining the best health of their members. To keep a family in healthy physical, mental, and spiritual condition, it is not necessary to have regular consultations or to receive any special treatment from a family doctor. The best natural method is the common traditional practice of gathering the family together regularly to eat meals that are well-prepared by the healthy central person of the household. Usually this position has been held by a woman who is mature physically and mentally. Through this practice the family is able to achieve the following benefits:

(1) Everyone's physical and mental conditions are thoroughly observed by each other and meals can be adjusted according to everyone's requirements. Special dishes may even be prepared for certain members of the family.

(2) Every member exchanges daily thoughts and experiences in intimate conversation.

(3) All family members are producing the same quality of blood by being nourished by the same quality of food, and therefore are sharing with one another the same dream and destiny.

Without such practice, there is no biological, psychological, and social unity, which is the essence of the family. The home becomes only an impersonal living place. People become disassociated especially when everyone eats in separate ways. Personalities and opinions begin to differ, eventually causing a lack of understanding and sympathy. Though there may be other contributing factors, the fundamental reason for the increase of conflicts, arguments, separation and divorce among married people and the disintegration of the family members, is the biological disagreement among these people.

Similarly, in community life, if the majority of people do not have the proper dietary practice with natural organic food prepared macrobiotically, there are constant repercussions. In such a community there is an increase in the number of sick people suffering both physically and mentally. Together with the decomposition of family life, many people become unable to support themselves, which results in the

---

Heart Diseases

The superior vena cava (A) and pulmonary artery (B) as well as the pulmonary vein are often clogged by the accumulation of heavy fat and cholesterol, along with tissue expansion in these arteries and veins. Also, the wall of the heart (C) accumulates hard fats which eventually penetrate to the tissues of the heart walls, resulting in immobility of the heart. Also, inharmonious coordination between right atrium and left atrium due to the expansion or contraction of a part of the heart as well as partial hardening of the heart tissues causes heart murmur and irregular beating. Furthermore, general enlargement of the heart caused by loosening of tissues causes abnormal blood pressure including hyper- and hypotension. All these heart troubles come from (1) animal food and other food containing heavy saturated fat, (2) sugar, honey, and other sweeteners causing formation of fatty acid and (3) excessive liquid, fruits, fruit juices, wine and other alcoholic beverages, loosening the elasticity of heart tissues.

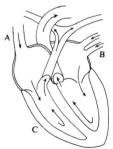

constant expansion of public welfare systems. Medical facilities as well as public insurance must continuously enlarge their scope. Psychological disorders among people require the construction not only of larger mental clinics but also of extensive legal systems and powerful bureaucracies.

The structure and operation of such societies is based upon fear and suspicion, insecurity and anxiety. Human relations become laden with distrust as people suffer from false, self-imposed delusions. Egocentric selfishness prevails over the community life with every member becoming defensive and protective of his private interests and benefits. To meet such circumstances, the community must produce systems of government and organized education which are more powerful, attempting to regulate and restrict everyone with rules and ethics. Training is geared toward standardization; everyone is taught the same concepts to meet the uniform set of requirements. Greater sickness of the community's people only leads to greater organization of the society. At the same time, the spreading physical and mental degeneration among the people causes rapid internal weakening of the society itself. Finally, replete with sick people, including its leaders, and economically unable to support itself, the community collapses.

C. *Biological Revolution*

In this twentieth century, our modern societies are rapidly declining from such basic biological causes. Modern preventive and protective measures are constantly increasing, yet proving ineffective:

(1)   Religious teachings are losing their influence on the people; ethical and moral codes and century-old traditions are no longer adaptable, with the result that there are no common principles and philosophies by which people may live.

(2)   Modern education has lost the spirit of respect for teachers and teachings, and love for the students, and no longer instills in the students the understanding of life.

(3)   Medical establishments are suffering from higher expenses, ineffective treatments, and an ever-increasing number of patients.

(4)   Families are decomposing rapidly; individual and social crimes are mounting.

In this modern crisis, all historical measures to change society whether spiritual and religious, social and educational, philosophical and scientific, or political and economic, are obsolete. Humanism such as in the Renaissance, revolution like that of France in 1789, declarations of freedom, as we see in the history of the United States, reformations as in Protestantism, ideologies such as Communism, concepts such as democracy, and technological works such as space travel—all are unable to save modern people from their rapid degeneration.

Although purification with oil was made by Abraham, baptism with water was done by John on the River Jordan, and salvation with the Holy Spirit was practiced by the early Christians, now is the time for the last and most fundamental method of purifying humanity and changing the destiny of mankind—biological renewal of our blood.

This biological change of humanity is the most peaceful revolution, not requiring any laws or doctrines, violence or mass movement. It is also the most universal revolution, able to prevail throughout the world, crossing over national, racial, ideological, religious, and cultural boundaries. It spreads from person to person, home to home, community to community, and country to country, beginning in every kitchen and ending in the realization of one peaceful world.

To reverse a course of degeneration to achieve one peaceful world is to secure the endless development of humanity. The new course follows this general progression:

(1)   Regaining the common-sense understanding about humanity, our origin and our future, our relations with the order of the universe, and its practical application in our daily lives.

(2)   Recovery of the wholesome quality of food through refomation of agriculture and traditional food processing methods.

(3)   World-wide distribution of these food products and their preparation according to macrobiotic principles.

(4)   Recovery of the physical and mental health of every person, family, and community through the above practices.

(5)   Development of a new orientation of society including education, culture, economy, and politics, from such a healthy biological foundation.

(6)   The dissolution of unnecessary and destructive defensive and protective measures through a gradual and natural elevation of consciousness from the basic stages of fear and insecurity.

(7)   The establishment of one world society within which everyone is able to enjoy health, freedom, and happiness by the gradual elimination of all discriminative boundaries.

2. World Governmental Organization

A.   Historical Review

From the beginning of written history, men have been continuously seeking a peaceful society. This desire has been felt not only among people who love peace, but also among those who have engaged in war in order to achieve peace. Even Alexander the Great and Genghis Khan, Napoleon and Hitler were inspired in the direction of war with the dream of establishing a peaceful unity among people. Plato's *Republic* (370 B.C.), Augustine's *The City of God* (A.D. 413), Thomas Moore's *Utopia* (1516), Campanella's *The City of the Sun* (1623), Hobbes's *Leviathan* (1651),

---

Resolution in the U.S. Congress on World Federal Government
(The following example is one of many similar resolutions designed and presented to the House of Representatives and the Senate in the United States Congress repeatedly after World War II.)
"The resolution, designed to put Congress on record in favor of strengthening and developing the United Nations, is as follows: '*Resolved by the House of Representatives* (*The Senate Concurring*), that it is the sense of the Congress that it should be a fundamental objective of the foreign policy of the United States to support and strengthen the United States and to seek its development into a world federation open to all nations with defined and limited powers adequate to preserve peace and prevent aggression through the enactment, interpretation, and enforcement of world law.' "
Congressional Record, Vol. 96, Part 13, p. A665 (Appendix), 81st Congress, 2nd Session—Jan. 3, 1950 to Feb. 28, 1950.

Kant's *Discourse on Perpetual Peace* (1795), and numerous other dreams of ideal and peaceful societies have been presented throughout history.

When World War I (1914–18) ended with great suffering and misery, the League of Nations was formed to avoid the possible destruction of future warfare. When the League collapsed and World War II (1939–45) brought greater destruction throughout the world, the United Nations was formed among the major modern countries to maintain international peace and security. In addition to such political efforts, there have been many international efforts through religious and humanitarian, economic and cultural cooperation. The world has definitely been moving towards an internationally organized society. Cooperative systems of mutual assistance have been bringing different nations and races, traditions and customs, cultures and ideologies toward world-wide unity. Such international cooperation now encompasses almost all domains, including communication, transportation, space exploration, the use of energy, financial investment, and problems of health and welfare.

However, despite this growing tendency towards the creation of a world society, several important problems remain to be solved in order to truly realize one peaceful world.

Political conflicts between liberal and communistic countries, economic conflicts between developed and undeveloped countries, religious conflicts between Catholics and Protestants, Christians and Moslems, old doctrines and new beliefs, cultural conflicts between theoretical sciences and aesthetic understanding, traditional conflicts between Western and Eastern customs, and many other such conflicts, are still causing difficulties and divisive thinking in the world today. Since 1945, serious attempts have been made to overcome these various conflicts—especially those involving national interests—by forming one world government. Among those who have contributed to this cause are Thomas Mann, Upton Sinclair, Norman Cousins, Albert Einstein, Robert Hutchins[1], Henry Osborne[2], and Edgar Gavaert[3] among Western thinkers, as well as Mahatma Gandhi, Jawaharlal Nehru, Toyohiko Kagawa[4], George Ohsawa, and others among Asian thinkers. During this period, proposals to establish a world federal government have been presented in the congresses of many countries, and it has been urged to adopt this goal as an objective of their international policies. Movements to establish world federal governments have consisted of two major currents, during the years between 1945 and 1955:

a. To amend the United Nations charter to develop a world federal government by limiting national sovereignty.

b. To form a world congress with the representatives of the people chosen in elections by the citizens of each country.

During the same period, more than fifty drafts of world constitutions were pro-

[1] Director of Ford Foundation
[2] British Member of Parliament
[3] Noted Belgian naturalist, artist and thinker
[4] Leading Christian leader and evangelist in Japan

posed by individuals, organizations, research groups, and other associations. Chicago University's special committee to draft a world constitution published its "Preliminary Draft of World Constitution." The world federal governments viewed by such proposals would be organized with political constitutions, similar to that of the United States. The world congress is proposed to have two houses: one house represented by every national government, and the other house composed of representatives elected by the people, probably one representative for each million of population.

B. *Limitations of the Proposed World Government*

A long-cherished dream of mankind has been the establishment of one world government, whether expressed as one world, one world community, world commonwealth, or world federation, and that dream has become more universally popular due to our vast technological development, including interplanetary space travel. However, even if such a world government or world federation were formed as a political and social structure, it would not be the ultimate solution for the happiness of mankind. A world community with a central government would be able to halt world-wide destruction and warfare, especially if the central government powerfully controlled all major destructive measures, including nuclear power. However, even with the formation of world government, many problems related to human happiness would remain unsolved:

(1) Halting warfare does not necessarily eliminate the cause of warfare. It would serve as an effective symptomatic treatment for the problems, but not as the cure of the underlying cause. Peace is not merely the absence of war; it is a state in which no cause for war exists. Such a state is possible when all conflicting factors are serving each other as complemental aids, and moreover, when no one thinks of war as a possible solution to any problem. In other words, peace can be realized only when people have no concept of war in their consciousness, a mentality not gained through public education or social training, but through the biological and psychological improvement of humanity. Simply speaking, when everyone reaches a physical and mental condition free of nightmares and delusions, peace in society is naturally realized. Any structural change of society, including the establishment of world government, does not serve to realize this true peace, if there is not also a biological and psychological improvement of humanity.

(2) Even if a world government were established, serving for political, economic and social unity, there would continuously be numerous physical and mental disorders in the form of various sicknesses, if a sound biological foundation were not also secured. Modern man would continue to degenerate and eventually the internal structure of such a world community would decompose by the weakening of human abilities. In the event any world program were designed along a course which would allow the possible decline of humanity—as demonstrated in modern national policies which have been producing environmental pollution, food contamination, and the energy crisis, as well as family dissolution and human distrust—the degeneration and unhappiness of humanity as a whole would be accelerated on a world-wide scale.

(3) If the world government were to adopt world education, it would tend to standardize all the people of the world according to regulated forms and concepts, hindering individual ingenuity and creativity. Especially if the entire world were organized with legal structures, human relations would become dominated by the concepts of contracts and laws instead of love, sympathy, and understanding. This tendency would stimulate the decline of human nature in the direction of mechanical living.

Without the biological and psychological revolution of humanity through the understanding of the order of nature and the law of the universe and through proper dietary practices suitable to the environment, any change of social, political, and economic systems including the establishment of a world federal government is merely symptomatic, and therefore temporary. Such systems would inevitably become ineffective and would eventually become harmful for the real happiness of mankind. The more powerful such systems are, the greater the danger is.

A dream of one peaceful world, or of one world government, is imperishable, but it can be achieved only through the development of humanity by biological, psychological, and spiritual improvement:

First, the elimination of all physical and mental-spiritual disorders by the establishment of the wholesome health of each individual;

Second, the elimination of all nightmares and delusions from human consciousness, through such improvements;

Third, the development of universal love and understanding among people, overcoming all differences of nationality and race, tradition and culture, belief and ideology, recognizing everyone as brothers and sisters of one great family of the universe.

By these steps, a united world will be realized in the natural course of the development of human society. There are no other ways to bring this about.[5]

C. Beyond National Boundaries

When we fly over the land, we see mountains, rivers, forests and fields, and we see no borderlines. When we voyage on the ocean, we see skies and clouds, water and waves, but we see no boundaries. All animals, all species spread across land and ocean. Why do we, mankind—particularly modern man—create limitations, and live within certain boundaries? If we saw this planet from a distance, far away in space, as if we were looking down from the window of a spacecraft, we would laugh at our folly in establishing national boundaries with the rigid concept of sovereignty.

What is a nation? A nation does not exist in nature and on this earth. A nation

---

Image of Forthcoming Peace
"The wolf shall dwell with the lamb: and the leopard shall lie down with the kid: the calf and the lion, and the sheep shall abide together, and a little child shall lead them. The calf and the bear shall feed: their young ones shall rest together: and the lion shall eat straw like the ox. And the suckling child shall play on the hole of the asp: and the weaned child shall thrust his hand into. the den of the basilisk. They shall not hurt, nor shall they kill in all my holy mountain, for the earth is filled with the knowledge of the Lord, as the covering waters of the sea."
The Old Testament, Isaiah, Ch. 11, 6–9.

exists only in a concept which we have come to believe through modern education, and we behave according to this learned concept. While no identification is required among all other species, modern man must carry a passport and visa as well as all other permits and identification papers. Beyond any doubt, we are limiting the space where we may live, and we are restricting our freedom of behavior. Before we are a citizen of any nation, we are citizens of the human race. Before our country is one of the existing nations, our country is this earth, this solar system, and this universe. National borderlines which have been designed for political reasons during the course of history should be gradually replaced by more natural territorial arrangements depending on differences in climatic and geographical conditions as well as in available food and dietary practices. Because of these factors, natural differences in people's physical and mental conditions arise, and therefore our many cultural and social varieties appear. Based on these differences, natural territorial arrangements would become evident. The future structure of the nation and its cultural, social and spiritual heritage should spring from its biological nature, and should not be imposed for any other reasons. Real sovereignty should not belong to any political and economic power wishing to demonstrate the independence of nations; but it lies in the physical and mental health of individual people, with sound spirit and consciousness, and in the law of nature and the order of the infinite universe, which are in no way indivisible and imperishable.

3. The Future World Community

The future world community should be designed and operated on the ideological ground that all human beings are brothers and sisters of one great family of the universe. World government should not be as political in nature as we have been experiencing in the modern orientation of national governments. The function of the world governmental organization should be one of education and service, and should not extend beyond that. As a matter of fact, all national governments should be developed to become educational and service organizations, gradually reducing their function of legal or authoritative enforcement.

A. World Fundamental Education
World organizations should serve the people of the world to gain an understanding of the order of the universe and the law of nature, and its relation with humanity. Every person should understand from where he has come and to where he shall go, and must orient his life according to his desire and ability.

(1) On the most elementary level, all people should learn how to keep their health and what to do when they become sick. They should have a knowledge of their daily food and should learn the effectiveness of appropriate dietary practices for their physical, mental, and spiritual development. They should also learn that they are primarily responsible for their own health and destiny.

(2) On the secondary level, they should learn the basic way of living, including cooking, sewing, housekeeping, gardening, and basic repairing. On this level they

should also understand how to take care of other people when they are sick, and should learn the spirit of love and care for other people.

On this secondary level, everyone should also master the primary ways of communication, including speaking, writing, calculating, and other expressions of our theoretical and aesthetic natures. They should read widely in all subjects and in many styles, including stories and poetry. They should experience physically and mentally through actual participation, the making of crafts, creative arts, gardening and housekeeping.

(3) At the following third level, all people should learn the spirit of respect to the elders, including parents and ancestors. The history of mankind also should begin to be presented, including specific personal family and community histories. Everyone's health should be maintained through active physical exercise, preferably interwoven with the daily life. Basic farming of the essential foods as well as all basic knowledge and techniques for life should be learned.

At this same level, everyone should be encouraged to observe and experience various natural phenomena, to know how those phenomena are changing in an orderly fashion according to the law of the universe. The antagonistic and complemental constitution of the endless universe should be revealed in simple and practical expression. The spirit of marvel at nature and the universe should be encouraged to grow. Knowledge should not be given, but rather everyone should be guided to discover for himself. The understanding of yin and yang is the tool to solve various questions and matters of wonder that everyone should have in mind. All possible artistic expressions should be encouraged.

(4) In the fourth level, pre-adolescent or early teenage education should be designed for both boys' and girls' common interests, but separate classes should also be arranged for their different interests. Boys should be given more physically- and socially-constructed training with emphasis on developing their courage and ambitions, while girls should be encouraged to develop more their sensitivity and understanding. Proper relations between man and woman should be well understood, with the aid of reasonable guidance. For both boys and girls, of course, there should be continuous encouragement for exploring and learning about human affairs and social events, as well as natural phenomena including the biological, psychological and spiritual realms, and the understanding of the earth, the solar system, and the celestial order.

Active life experiences, including the learning of technological skills as well as involvement in social life and human relations, should be arranged, in addition to intellectual and aesthetic studies. Common sense based upon the universal consciousness of the brother- and sisterhood of all mankind should be developed on this level.

(5) From the following fifth level, the latter period of adolescence, everyone should be given the opportunity of starting to choose his major path of learning according to his own interests. From this level on, some people would follow a more academic direction, some more technical training, and others a more professional orientation. However, everyone should be continuously encouraged to make their own inventive discoveries and creations, and to find answers to their own

questions. At this level everyone should gain the profound understanding that the order which is working in our body and mind is also working in human relations and in society, and the very same order is also working in all phenomena throughout the universe. At this level, also, respect to all ancestors of mankind and love to all offspring should be confirmed.

(6)   From the next, sixth, level—post-adolescence and the late teenage years— everyone should be free to pursue his or her own interests regardless of subject and of whether they learn through intellectual studies or through actual experiences. Throughout this period, they should be guided to reflect for themselves, to judge themselves, and to discover who they are, what dream they should pursue and how they should play throughout their lives. Not only the physical, material world, but also the spiritual and invisible world should be understood through their own study and experience.

(7)   At the seventh stage, everyone should be encouraged to express his own discoveries, inventions, and assumptions to the public, either in writing or in speech, and to demonstrate this acquired experience in public in any manner he or she wishes to choose. The imitation or copying of previously existing ideas and thoughts should be discouraged. When such original creations, expressed in any manner, are performed well, it is considered that education is completed. There should be no definite time of graduation and there should be no requirement to remain in the educational system after the fourth level.

Comprehensively speaking, the principles of world education are:

(a)   Everyone is free to orient his life according to his own dream;

(b)   Everyone should be creative and inventive, in his own search;

(c)   Everyone and every phenomenon is related as manifestations of this great family of the infinite universe;

(d)   The spirit of harmony, respect, and love is the essence of individual health and of the development of humanity as a whole.

B.   World Public Service

Another major function of world government or organization, besides world education, is world public service. This service consists of three main aspects: (1) public utility service, (2) public health service, and (3) natural agriculture.

(1)   *The public utility service* offers all conveniences necessary for healthy living, including world communications, transportation, construction of world-wide utility systems, and distribution of necessary materials and natural resources. Public services designed for territorial and national needs should be primarily responsible for such local services and functions, but world-wide services should be offered equally to everyone through the world public service.

(2)   *The public health service* includes not only the maintenance and protection of people's health from physical and mental disorders, but also the nourishment of all sorts of criminal people according to the proper dietary practices, in order to make them physically and mentally sound. All crimes are the manifestation of physical and mental sickness. Any legal compulsory punishment imposed upon those who have committed any crimes or other socially undesirable behavior, should

be replaced by proper nutritional care and mental education.

The need for medical care and facilities would become naturally reduced, except for some cases such as emergencies, as public education develops the proper dietary practices among all people, allowing adaptation to the natural environment. At the same time, proper dietary practices would cause a decrease in psychological disorders, resulting in the drastic decrease of violence, hatred, prejudice, and greed. Society would automatically become more peaceful and yet, more energetic in the pursuit of constructive progress. Pharmaceutical care and various insurance programs would naturally lose their value. Together with proper education, the world health service would become, in a sense, the most powerful factor in maintaining a peaceful society.

(3) *Natural agriculture.* The physical, mental, and spiritual health of the world's people depends mostly upon their daily practice of proper diet according to the order of the universe. The macrobiotic way of dietary practice suggests the following principles:

a. Agricultural products should be chosen according to the territorial environment in order that the people consuming them may properly adapt to their surroundings. In the case of continents which have little geographic and climatic variety, as in North America, the food that we eat should be produced approximately within a 500-mile radius. In the case of other continents or areas such as Western Europe and India, which have more geographic and climatic variety, this radius should be decreased to about 200 miles, or in proportion to the degree of variety. In the case of islands such as the Far Eastern and Northern European Isles, this radius should be further decreased, possibly to 100 miles, because of the richness in the variety of geographic and climatic conditions.

b. Agriculture should be conducted according to the practices of natural-organic cultivation, avoiding the use of any chemically produced fertilizers, pesticides and insecticides. During the process of human evolution over millions of years, chemicals were not applied in the production of food—until only a short time ago, the early part of the 20th century. Because of the use of thousands of varieties of chemicals, which are mostly extremely yin, agricultural products have become larger in appearance and volume. However, they have lost their strength, vitality, and rich taste, as well as their compact organic structure. By eating those products, we modern men and women have been rapidly weakening our physical and mental conditions and developing more yin tendencies. The abundant use of chemical fertilizer further depletes one of our most important natural resources—the elements in the soil— and adversely affects the life of the microorganisms in the soil which are serving for the healthy growth of plants.

We should return as soon as possible to the natural, organic methods of cultivation which have been traditionally performed throughout the world for many centuries.

c. However, in order to not only maintain and protect our health from various modern degenerative diseases, but also to develop further our health and well-being, physically, mentally, and spiritually as a strong human species, our agriculture should be further developed from natural-organic cultivation to an even more natural agriculture. The objective of this natural agriculture is to restore artificially cultivated grains, beans, and vegetables to their natural, wild character.

This natural agriculture is based upon the understanding that man has evolved through natural processes out of his environment, including the vegetable world. Man is a manifestation of the environmental conditions; it is not his function to change his environment. When we start to think that we should regulate our food by changing the quality of the plants or of the environment, this egocentric view makes an unnatural separation between man and his environment. By allowing the food to return from its present cultivated quality to its more natural and wild quality, we would be able to restore our true humanity—our most suitable condition, and our ability to adapt to the environment. Therefore, this new agriculture requires the gradual decrease of human participation in the cultivation of food, finally reaching a state in which the less we participate, the better the products are.

The practical method of this natural agriculture has the following principles:

a. *Non-Weeding:* Weeds and vegetable plants naturally occur together. The practice of weeding reduces the natural tilling of the soil which is done by the roots of various weeds, and decreases the living microorganisms which normally thrive among the roots of the weeds. The healthy growth of weeds is beneficial to the flourishing of various vegetable plants.

In agricultural cultivation, desirable weeds are the smaller varieties such as clover and many other shorter, softer weeds. It would be necessary to replace the larger weeds with these more desirable kinds.

b. *Non-Tilling:* If weeds are removed, the soil is not tilled by the usual natural process, and human labor for tilling becomes necessary. When such tilled soil receives rainfall, it tends to become harder, requiring even further labor for tilling. On the other hand, if we leave the desirable weeds in the field, thereby accomplishing natural tilling, these weeds also help to hold water from the rainfalls, and keep the soil more suitably moist. Artificially-tilled soil cannot keep such moist conditions for a long period.

c. *Non-Fertilizing:* Because of weeding and tilling, the soil produces only those vegetables which are planted, and large spaces are left open between the plants. Fertilizers must be brought in from outside, and applied to the land in order to maintain a condition rich in nutrients. However, if weeds are allowed to grow on the land, they replenish the soil when they die, securing the same soil conditions for the coming year. Furthermore, if we return the unused portion of harvested plants to the land, these would further enrich the soil, serving to maintain the original soil conditions.

d. *Non-Spraying:* If we cultivate only a single species of plant in an area, we often receive an invasion of insects, worms, and animals which are attracted to that particular species. Of course, this is mainly due to the practice of weeding and to the practice of mono-cultivation—cultivation of a single species in one area. However, if we keep the land covered with weeds or various species of plants, and if we plant several species of vegetables which differ from each other in character—for example, planting not all root vegetables or all leafy vegetables but a mixture of the two—such invasions are minimized. In nature, there is no place where only a single species of plant is growing; there are always several different species growing cooperatively. Development from mono-cultivation to poly-cultivation is essential for natural agriculture.

e. *Non-Seeding:* At harvest time, we should not take all of the products; we should leave 10%–20% unharvested, growing upon the land. These remaining plants produce seeds which eventually are scattered over the land, and from these seeds new plants start to grow. When we repeat this process over several years, seeding by human labor becomes unnecessary, and labor would be needed only to thin out excessive growth. In the case of cereal grains, this method may not be applicable, particularly in smaller fields; but other plants, including most varieties of vegetables, can be left to their own natural cycles of growth.

f. *Non-Pruning:* In order to insure the natural growth and development of any plant, especially tree plants producing fruits and flowers, we should avoid artificial pruning. All plants grow their branches and leaves according to certain laws of nature. When we interfere by artificial trimming, cutting and pruning, the plants can no longer maintain their natural quality. Of course, this results in the production of an unnatural quality of fruits and flowers. To our human eyes, pruned trees may appear more beautiful or symmetrical, but they are actually deformed and un-balanced in the eyes of nature. A natural quality of plants produces a natural quality of humanity, and an unnatural quality of plants produces an unnatural, weak humanity.

Generally speaking, natural agriculture is the agriculture which can bring about the recovery of modern civilized humanity, which is degenerating rapidly at this time due to its physical, mental and spiritual disorders. When our daily food becomes naturally strong, not only our physical health but also our spiritual development advances without limit. Our psychological ability, including the faculties of telepathy, foresight, imagination, insight, and so-called extra-sensory perception, begins to develop with the natural quality of food. The method of cooking as well as the volume of food required would change greatly. We begin to truly appreciate the natural taste of foods with their wholesome richness; the use of artificial flavoring would become unnecessary, and the use of a little sea salt and vegetable oil in cooking would satisfy our desire. Natural agriculture is the gate opening into the garden of paradise, which we lost long before our written history began.

4. New Principles of Economy

When we consider all living species other than our modern civilized people, we see that all animals running in the fields, all birds flying in the sky, and all fishes swim-ming in the waters, are always playing; they do not work. When we reflect how the human race began on this earth some millions of years ago, we wonder whether it is really necessary for the continuation of our life, to continue to work in such a regulated manner as organized in our modern society. It is common understanding that we have to work in order to support our living, especially when we would like to enjoy our freedom. Do we really need to work? If so, why is it only necessary for modern man? Or, if not, what is wrong in the orientation of our modern society?

When we were born as infants, did we expect that the greater part of our adult life would be dedicated to working for our livelihood, without doing what we really want to do? Have we come from the infinite universe to this earth, manifesting as human beings, in order to learn how to work, to engage every day in regulated activities, and to retire from such engagement at the age of 60 or 65, followed soon after by our death? How many people in the modern world are really enjoying their lives and doing what they want to do? Were we born to work, or were we born to play? For what purpose is our life? If we are not enjoying wholehearted play from morning to night, is it really worthwhile to continue our lives, even for a few years? One of the essential problems all modern men and women are confronting is whether we are doing, every day, what we really want to do.

The principles of economy which are universally applicable in human life are found in the understanding of what we are and what the universe is. We, modern men and women, like all other natural phenomena, are manifestations of this infinite universe. The order of the universe is also reflected in the principles of economy, with which every modern man needs to manage his life. These principles can be comprehensively expressed as follows:

A. One Grain—Ten Thousand Grains

This universe is constantly expanding, as modern astronomical research is revealing. Infinite expansion is the fundamental nature of this infinite universe itself. Within this universe, therefore, every phenomenon tends to expand, differentiate, and reproduce endlessly. The law of natural production is constant creation. One grain, if it falls on the proper soil, produces hundreds of grains. They, in turn, produce hundreds of thousands of grains, and they further produce hundreds of millions of grains.

The principle of economy which we should use in our administration and operation is, therefore, endless production and endless distribution. For this, we should use natural methods as much as possible, and we should minimize artificial efforts, because there are no factors more powerful than nature and the universe. When we intend to apply our human technology to accelerate and reinforce natural powers, it tends to disturb the entire peaceful movement of natural cycles, which in turn results in the destruction of our health and the existence of the human species—or even the existence of this earth itself.

B. The Capital of Our Economy

The fundamental resource or capital of our economy is neither financial power nor the productive ability of machinery and equipment. These are secondary factors —the means to operate production and distribution. The real capital is: (1) the physical, mental and spiritual health of all individual people of the world, and (2) the natural forces and environmental conditions, including the earth, solar system, and the universe. Therefore, if human health deteriorates and the natural environment is damaged and depleted through some so-called economic enterprises, as we are experiencing increasingly in this century, these operations are in reality anti-economy: against the principles of economy for everyone's well-being and universal peace.

Before anything else, humanity should be healthy and sound, for which macrobiotic principles and the practice of proper diet should be applied everywhere in the world. This will secure the fundamental capital for all kinds of economic operations.

At the same time, sources of energy should not be sought in the deposited resources of the earth, which are limited and therefore exhaustible. We should seek energy and power not within the earth, but among the forces which have created and are moving the earth, including solar energy, electromagnetic power in the solar system, vibrations, waves, and rays coming without limit from the universe towards this earth.

C.   Principles of Operation

The operation of any economic enterprise should be conducted consciously with the understanding of yin and yang, the laws of balance and harmony. Balance and harmony should be maintained between (1) the universe and the earth, (2) biological life and the environment, (3) all animal and vegetable life, and the human species, (4) world human production and territorial needs, and (5) material wealth and individual well-being. These five major areas of balance and harmony should be carefully considered in the design and operation of all economic enterprises. At present, the driving force of modern economy is mainly the pursuit of material wealth, convenience, and comfort. Because of this narrow, limited orientation, human well-being, including physical and mental health, is in danger, in spite of economic prosperity. Environmental conditions, all other biological species, and the existence of the earth itself are approaching a critical stage.

The supply of food and basic living necessities should be arranged within each territory in order to adapt harmoniously to the natural environment, along the principles of self-support and self-sufficiency.

All other additional materials and facilities can be traded widely and freely throughout the world, in order to share intellectual understanding and aesthetic experience, as well as the benefits of world civilization.

We are confronting at the present time a reorientation of all economic principles which we have been using for centuries, by examining whether these principles and methods of economy are really serving constructively for the well-being of mankind. The ideas of Adam Smith, John Maynard Keynes, Karl Marx, as well as other theories of capitalism, socialism and communism, are not necessarily based upon the understanding of the principles of the universe and of what is needed for the health and well-being of every person. Economic systems and structures should develop more naturally, rather than being constructed from conceptual theories, as our consciousness develops towards the recognition of our status as brothers and sisters living together on this earth. Economic systems should be gradually reoriented and developed in the nature of family systems, whether on a world, territorial or small family scale. Economy following the nature of the family is to be based upon love and respect for everyone and for every other species, and for all environmental conditions including nature, the earth, and the universe.

The world community would fall into chaos unless we proceed with biological, psychological, and spiritual revolution by means of the proper way of life based upon macrobiotic principles. The world community will become peaceful and flourish if everyone in the world establishes his health and well-being by applying the understanding of the order of the universe. It is up to us, whether we are able to establish one peaceful world which we can pass on, generation to generation, to all our offspring.

From Here to Eternity

A. The Spiral of History

The development of world history has described an inward-moving logarithmic spiral, alternating between the yang periods of the concentration of territorial power, and the yin periods of universalization by idea. Each half-orbit of the spiral represents one of our historical periods. Each period is approximately one-third as long as the previous period. In other words, each period changes with three times the speed of the previous age. The change of society as well as the development of technology and consciousness is accelerating logarithmically.

Fig. 34   The Spiral of History

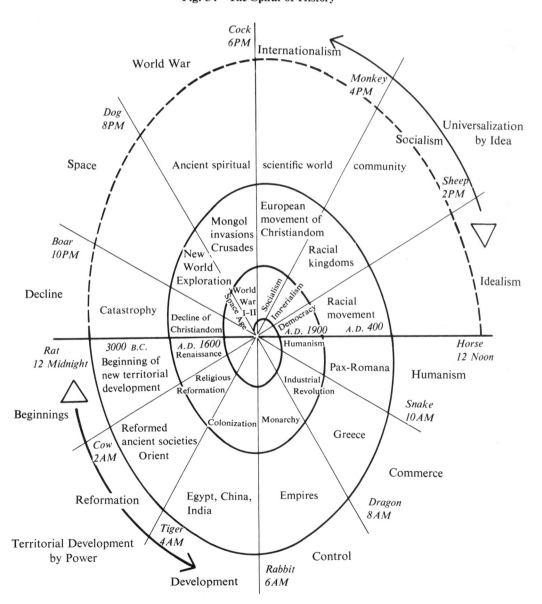

At the same time, the use of fire has increased in a similar ratio, as the source of fire and energy changed from wood to charcoal, charcoal to coal, coal to petroleum, petroleum to electricity, electricity to nuclear power. The increasing use of energy also accelerates the change of human society in the historical spiral.

(1) *The Age of the Ancient Spiritual and Scientific World Community*

The ancient world community which shared megalithic stone culture and similar cosmologies here and there throughout the world, ended by catastrophic changes in nature along with the decline of humanity, up to approximately 3000 B.C.

(2) *The Ancient Age*

Written history began around 3000 B.C. with the beginning of new territorial developments succeeding the heritage remaining from the preceding ancient world community. Such new developments occurred in northern China, northwest India, Mesopotamia, the Upper Nile and Mediterranean regions, as well as the north-western part of South America. This age was governed by political, social and economic power in the formation of empires and ended about A.D. 400, around the time of the collapse of Rome in Western European history.

(3) *The Medieval Age*

The beginning of this period was guided more by religious and ideological powers, namely Christianity in the case of Europe, including the formation of racial kingdoms, such as the Germans, Saxons, Normans and others. Two notable world wars, the Mongol invasions from east to west, and the Crusades moving from west to east, occurred during this time. This period ended with the exploration and discovery of new territories in Africa, Asia and Australia, followed by the decline of Christiandom in Europe.

(4) *The Modern Age*

This new age began with the Renaissance around A.D. 1600. Religious reformations began, including various forms of Protestantism in Europe. In Asia, reformed teachings of Confucianism, Buddhism and other religious doctrines also arose during this period. Various areas of the world were colonized by western powers. Such monarchies as the Hapsburgs, Bourbons and Romanovs flourished; however, this was followed by the rise of the bourgeoisie, and soon after, by the political and industrial revolution and the humanistic movement, which developed toward democracy. This period ended in the early 1900s.

(5) *The Recent Age*

In the early 20th century, the new age began with the flourishing of democracy and the formation of modern nations. Imperialistic, socialistic and communistic movements developed on the international scale. International society started to be formed, and at the same time, World Wars I and II were experienced. Soon after the world wars, the exploration of space began—towards the moon, Venus, and other celestial bodies. However, this age has been drawing to a close with the decomposition of families, religious and spiritual authorities, and educational systems, as well as the decline of human health—physical, mental, and spiritual.

(6) *The Present Age*

In this latter part of the 20th century, we are beginning a new age—the last half-century before the historical spiral reaches its center. In this short period, all aspects of human affairs—religious and ideological, political and economic, social and cultural, individualistic and universal, liberal and conservative, warlike and peaceful, Eastern and Western, material and spiritual, and all other factors—would gather. This age is the most confused, complicated, and condensed period which mankind has ever experienced in its history. During this period, many changes will take place, and most conventional systems will collapse. Many millions of people will also suffer with various physical and mental disorders.

(7) *The End of Material Civilization*

Following the present age, the last stage of our long human history, which has been oriented by centripetal tendencies—following an inward spirallic path—will reach its end, as the center of the historical spiral is reached. Modern civilization as a whole will end tragically either through world-wide destruction by warfare, or by the total degeneration of humanity. However, at the same time, a new orientation of civilization will arise among those people who have individually reoriented their way of life according to the laws of nature and the order of the universe. Through their understanding and efforts, the construction of a new healthy and peaceful world will begin, by the unification of all antagonistic factors of human affairs. This we may describe as the establishment of world federal government, or the beginning of spiritual civilization, which will be directed by centrifugal development, moving from the center of our historical spiral towards the periphery, forming an outward-directed spiral. In this new spiritual civilization, the biological, psychological and spiritual health of every person is of fundamental importance, and all political, economic, ideological and cultural systems will be built more naturally upon that foundation.

After the beginning of the course of spiritual civilization, we, all of mankind, would enjoy one healthy and peaceful world, which will be generally accomplished about 2,000 years later. This world of spiritual civilization would continue further for nearly 10,000 years, until again it will decline and change its course toward material civilization: yin changing to yang, yang changing to yin, repeating eternally. Prosperity changes to poverty, poverty to prosperity. Materialism inevitably changes into spiritualism, but spiritualism, at its extreme height, will also inevitably turn into materialism.

Knowing the endless principles of the infinite order of the universe, we, mankind, shall maintain our status, always in health and sound condition, by meeting any changes of the trends of civilization, as well as any changes of the natural environment.

The understanding of the infinite order of the universe and the practice of daily life according to this understanding is the key for the endless happiness of everyone.

B. Everlasting Life

We have come from infinity. We have manifested ourselves, taking the course of physicalization and materialization of life. At the terminus of this course, we were conceived with our parents' reproductive cells, the egg (yang) and sperm (yin). This is the beginning of our return to our origin: the infinite universe. In this returning course, we dephysicalize and spiritualize ourselves, taking the expanding centri-

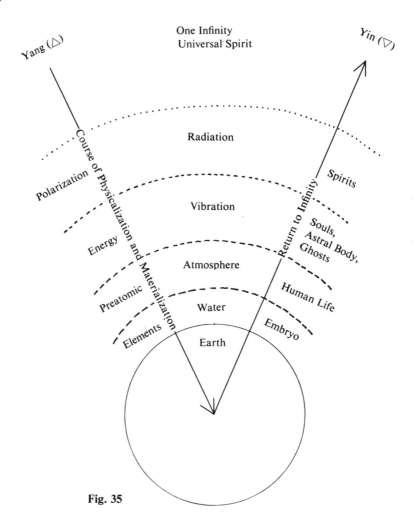

Fig. 35

fugal direction.

Our embryonic life was in a world of water in the mother's uterus, a small, dark world. In this world we created our protoplasmic body, the organism composed of cells, to prepare for the next life.

From there, we emerged, discarding the placenta and umbilical cord, into a new world surrounded in air. The far larger and brighter space within which we play is the entire surface of the earth. This world alternates between brightness and darkness, day and night. In this world, we continue to develop our protoplasmic body for the period of approximately twenty years.

Do we stop our development at that point, or do we continue our development of different qualities other than the physical body? We continue to develop unceasingly our emotional, intellectual, social, ideological, and universal consciousness together with the constant refinement of our physical qualities. We develop the bioplasmic body—our electromagnetic constitution which deals with vibrations and waves of consciousness.

When this bioplasmic body matures, in the same way that we transferred our-selves from the world of water to the world of air, we transfer our life to the world of vibration, in the form of bioplasm, leaving the protoplasmic body behind us. The world of vibration is far greater in space and far brighter, with no darkness. Consciousness is continued in this new world, which is usually called the spiritual world. The communication of consciousness is conducted not only in the spiritual world alone, but also between the spiritual world and the human world. The spatial dimension of this vibrational world covers the entire sphere of the solar system as one unit.

However, as we know, if the embryonic life in the mother's uterus is not properly nourished, a miscarriage, early birth, deformation or retardation arises, and infants who are born with these conditions must suffer in this human world. Similarly, if our nourishment in this air world is not proper, the result is deformation or retarda-tion in the physical, mental, and spiritual conditions, and during this life period we have to die unnaturally, probably because of sickness, accident, or other undesirable causes. This results in an unexpected, immature birth into the next, spiritual world. And such immature birth in that world causes us to suffer in darkness even though the world is full of light. In such cases, attachment and delusion of consciousness to this world makes these spirits wander among human society, often manifesting as ghosts.

In the event that nourishment is proper in this air world, and we have refined our physical, mental, and spiritual vibration to a level of maturity sufficient to be born into the next, vibrational world, our death is natural and spiritual. If we are born through such spiritual death into the next world, we enjoy a large dimension of free consciousness with spiritual happiness. Furthermore, after we accomplish the next life by the maturing of our spiritual quality, we further proceed to a higher and more universal plane, dissolving the vibrational body into waves and rays. This world is far larger, covering the entire dimension of this galaxy. From this stage, our life further continues and returns through changing ourselves into the infinite speed of motion, and eventually becomes one with the universal consciousness of infinity.

Our life is eternal, though our human life is ephemeral. Our dream is endless, though our human desires are finite. The will of life, the order of the infinite uni-verse, is boundless, though our human works are in vain. Living with our eternal life, changing ourselves constantly, manifesting ourselves into various forms, is our play in this universe. Our freedom is to change ourselves to adapt to the environ-ment, and to continue to develop endlessly.

Happiness is the endless realization of our infinite dream.

appendix

Memory and Spiritual Consciousness

As we have physicalized ourselves through the orbiting spiral of the universe into our present human status, we are a manifestation of infinity—past and future. Our physical-mental-spiritual manifestation is itself a condensed form of the memory which we have experienced from the beginningless beginning of this infinite universe. When we start to purify ourselves through proper dietary practice, we begin to clarify the delusions and cloudiness of our present consciousness along with the healing of our present physical disorders. As we progress to purify our physical-mental conditions, we further clarify older delusions and confusions which we experienced some years ago. At the same time our memory goes back to that period, recalling nature, people, and incidents experienced at that time. When we continue our purification, we further heal much older sicknesses hiding in the depths of our body, and also we recall experiences we had at that time. When we continue our purification over a seven-year period our cleansing reaches the physical-mental disorders of our infancy and early childhood. Memory further continues to go back, and when we continue to practice the macrobiotic way of life over 15 years, our consciousness goes back towards the plant kingdom, the earth and various celestial worlds, and we feel as if we ourselves are those phenomena, by developing our understanding and sympathy towards them. Thus, our memory goes back to the infinite universe itself after more than 20 years' practice of the macrobiotic way of life. Memory is equal to consciousness, and without memory there is no judgment. Universal consciousness is naturally developed by our own memory of the infinite universe. When our consciousness reaches this stage, we start to foresee our future, because our future life evolves within the infinite universe. Thus, universal consciousness melts past and future into one. The past is equal to the future. Memory is equal to dream. Eternal memory is eternal dream, and vice versa.

Remarks on Birth Control

Self-reflection is to use our own higher consciousness to observe, review, examine, and judge our thoughts and behavior which are motivated by our lower consciousnesses. We evaluate sensory and emotional conduct by our intellectual social judgment. We evaluate our intellectual and social conduct by our ideological and supreme judgment. When our memory goes back to our infinite origin and our endless dream becomes one with beginningless memory, our universal consciousness can orient all our thought and conduct with no mistake. When all our life is guided by our own universal consciousness—highest judgment, we are entirely free, knowing past and future. The more we reflect upon ourselves, the higher we become. When we become highest, our life manifests in the spirit of endless giving: one grain—ten thousand grains, along with the infinitely expanding universe. Ask yourself every day:

(1) Did I eat properly today, and did I chew well? (Biological reflection)
(2) Did I think of my parents and elders today, with love and respect? (Social reflection)
(3) Did I happily greet everyone today? (Psychological reflection)
(4) Did I marvel today at the wonders of nature? (Ideological reflection)
(5) Did I thank everyone and appreciate whatever I experienced today? (Comprehensive reflection)

These five are self-reflections that we should practice every day, regardless of our age, throughout our lives. This is the spirit of macrobiotic life.

General Appendix

DIETARY GOALS FOR UNITED STATES

Prepared by the Staff of the
Select Committee on Nutrition
and Human Needs
United States Senate
January, 1977
(*Excerpt From U.S. SENATE REPORT*)

Foreword

The purpose of this report is to point out that the eating patterns of this century represent as critical a public health concern as any now before us.

We must acknowledge and recognize that the public is confused about what to eat to maximize health. If we as a government want to reduce health costs and maximize the quality of life for all Americans, we have an obligation to provide practical guides to the individual consumer as well as set national dietary goals for the country as a whole.

Such an effort is long over-due. Hopefully, this study will be a first major step in that direction.

GEORGE MCGOVERN
Chairman

PART I
DIETARY GOALS FOR THE UNITED STATES

Introduction

During this century, the composition of the average diet in the United States has changed radically. Complex carbohydrates—fruit, vegetables and grain products—which were the mainstay of the diet, now play a minority role. At the same time, fat and sugar consumption have risen to the point where these two dietary elements alone now comprise at least 60 percent of total caloric intake, an increase of 20 percent since the early 1900's.[1]

In the view of doctors and nutritionists consulted by the Select Committee, these and other changes in the diet amount to a wave of malnutrition—of both over- and under-consumption—that may be as profoundly damaging to the nation's health as the widespread contagious diseases of the early part of the century.

The over-consumption of fat, generally, and saturated fat in particular, as well as cholesterol, sugar, salt and alcohol have been related to six of the ten leading causes of death:

---

[1] The food supply estimates are based on Department of Agriculture data showing the amounts of food that "disappear" into civilian channels. These figures, while not on an ingested basis, provide the best current measure of food use.

heart disease, cancer, cerebrovascular disease, diabetes, arteriosclerosis and cirrhosis of the liver.

In his testimony at the Select Committee's July 1976 hearings on the relationship of diet to disease, Dr. D. Mark Hegsted of Harvard School of Public Health, said:

> I wish to stress that there is a great deal of evidence and it continues to accumulate, which strongly implicates and, in some instances, proves that the major causes of death and disability in the United States are related to the diet we eat. I include coronary artery disease which accounts for nearly half of the deaths in the United States, several of the most important forms of cancer, hypertension, diabetes and obesity as well as other chronic diseases.

The over-consumption of food in general has become a major public health problem. In testimony at the same hearings, Dr. Theodore Cooper, Assistant Secretary for Health, estimated that about 20 percent of all adults in the United States "are overweight to a degree that may interfere with optimal health and longevity."

At the same time, current dietary trends may also be leading to malnutrition through under-nourishment. Fats and sugar are relatively low in vitamins and minerals. Consequently, diets reduced to control weight and/or save money, but which are high in fat and sugar, are likely to lead to vitamin and mineral deficiencies. As will be discussed later, low-income people may be particularly susceptible to inducements to consume high-fat/high-sugar diets.

In testimony before the Select Committee in 1972, Dr. George Briggs, professor of nutrition at the University of California, Berkeley, estimated, based on a study by the Department of Agriculture, that improved nutrition might cut the nation's health bill by one-third. The Department of Health, Education and Welfare's *Forward Plan for Health, FY 1978–82*, reports that health care expenditures in the United States in Fiscal Year 1975 totalled about $118.5 billion and predicts the cost could exceed $230 billion by Fiscal Year 1980.

Beyond the monetary saving, it is obvious then that improved nutrition also offers the potential for prevention of vast suffering and loss of productivity and creativity.

One in three men in the United States can be expected to die of heart disease or stroke before age 60 and one in six women. It is estimated that 25 million suffer from high blood pressure and that about 5 million are afflicted by diabetes mellitus.[2]

Given the wide impact on health that has been traced to the dietary trends outlined, it is imperative, as a matter of public health policy, that consumers be provided with authoritative dietary guidelines or goals that will encourage the most healthful selection of foods.

Such goals may be controversial. First, they must be based primarily on epidemiological evidence, findings of associations between certain dietary factors and incidence of disease. In addition, it would be helpful to base these goals on more current data on food consumption and health in the United States. Unfortunately, the nutrition surveys being conducted by the Departments of Agriculture, and Health, Education and Welfare will not report findings until 1978 at the earliest. It is also doubtful that the surveys, because of their structures, timing and lack of funding and coordination, will be able to make useful correlations between food consumption patterns and health. Finally, regardless of epidemio-

---

[2] Statistics from reports and testimony presented to the Select Committee's National Nutrition Policy hearings, June 1974, appearing in National Nutrition Policy Study, 1974, Pt. 6, June 21, 1974, heart disease, p. 2,633; high blood pressure, p. 2,529; diabetes, p. 2,523.

logical findings and survey results there will be honest professional disagreement over prescribed action.

Marc LaLonde, Canada's Minister of National Health and Welfare, speaks to this kind of problem in *A New Perspective on the Health of Canadians*, published in 1974:

> Even such a simple question as whether one should severely limit his consumption of butter and eggs can be a subject of endless scientific debate.
>
> Faced with conflicting scientific opinions of this kind, it would be easy for health educators and promotors to sit on their hands; it certainly makes it easy for those who abuse their health to find a real "scientific" excuse.
>
> But many of Canada's health problems are sufficiently pressing that action has to be taken even if all scientific evidence is not in.

Based on (1) testimony presented to the Select Committee in its July 1976 hearings on the relationship of diet to disease and its 1974 National Nutrition Policy hearings, (2) guidelines established by governmental and professional bodies in the United States and at least eight other nations (Appendix A), and (3) a variety of expert opinion, the following dietary goals are recommended for the United States. Although genetic and other individual differences mean that these guidelines may not be applicable to all, there is substantial evidence indicating that they will be generally beneficial.

United States Dietary Goals

1. Increase carbohydrate consumption to account for 55 to 60 percent of the energy (caloric) intake.

FIGURE 1.

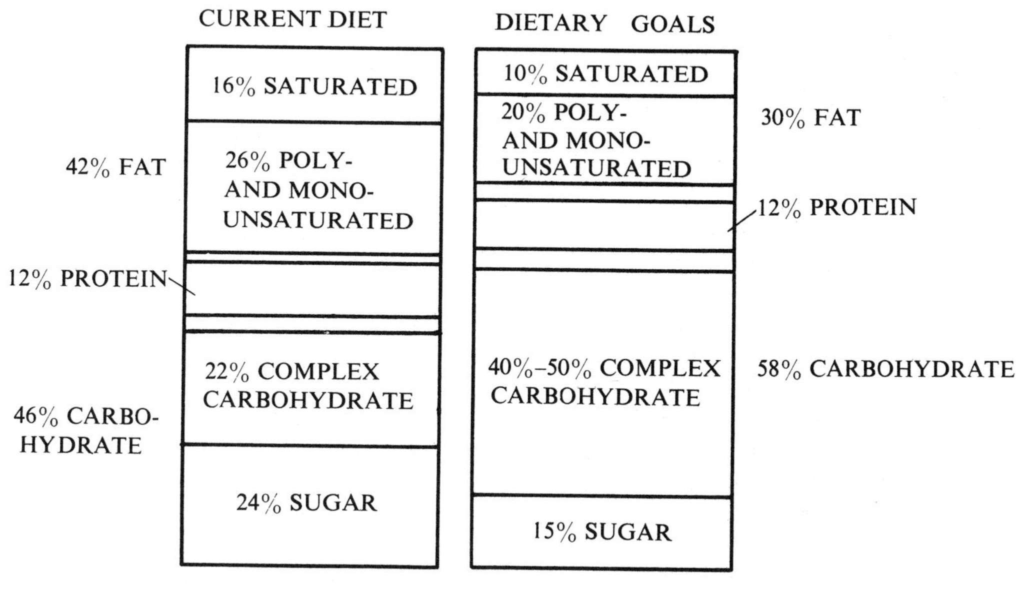

Sources for current diet: *Changes in Nutrients in the U.S. Diet Caused by Alterations in Food Intake Patterns.* B. Friend. Agricultural Research Service. U.S. Department of Agriculture. 1974. Proportions of saturated versus unsaturated fats based on unpublished Agricultural Research Service data.

2. Reduce overall fat consumption from approximately 40 to 30 percent of energy intake.
3. Reduce saturated fat consumption to account for about 10 percent of total energy intake; and balance with poly-unsaturated and mono-unsaturated fats, which should account for about 10 percent of energy intake each.
4. Reduce cholesterol consumption to about 300 mg. a day.
5. Reduce sugar consumption by almost 40 percent to account for about 15 percent of total energy intake.
6. Reduce salt consumption by about 50–85% to approximately 3 grams a day.

The goals are expressed graphically in Figure 1.

The Goals Suggest the Following
Changes in Food Selection and Preparation

1. Increase consumption of fruits and vegetables and whole grains.
2. Decrease consumption of meat and increase consumption of poultry and fish.
3. Decrease consumption of foods high in fat and partially substitute poly-unsaturated fat for saturated fat.
4. Substitute non-fat milk for whole milk.
5. Decrease consumption of butterfat, eggs and other high cholesterol sources.
6. Decrease consumption of sugar and foods high in sugar content.
7. Decrease consumption of salt and foods high in salt content.

A Historical Review of the Macrobiotic Movement in North America

The principle and practice of the macrobiotic way of life has been a universal tradition in every culture of mankind for unknown centuries. It has been applied for individual health and freedom as well as social peace and happiness. In the modern age, it has been recovered from traditional Oriental philosophy and culture, including Oriental medicine and religions.

During the period that Western thought and civilization began to be introduced and widely practiced in Oriental countries, these traditional Oriental philosophies and cultures subsided in nearly all domains. Western education became the official education, and promoted Western medicine. All political, economic, and social systems were changed to this new trend. In the middle of this huge current of westernization, however, there were some people who had studied Oriental traditions and a few. others who were attempting to synthesize both Oriental and Western thought. Among them are Sagen Ishizuka (石塚左玄) and his associates who formulated the dietary approach to various sicknesses, and learning from them, George Ohsawa began his studies.

George Ohsawa and his associates tried to see the essence of ancient Oriental cosmology as a basis for the solution of the problems of health and peace. Through their applications of diet, some hundreds of thousands of Japanese people received benefits until the time of World War II, recovering their health from various sicknesses. Passing through the most difficult period of the last world war, when he was in prison due to his anti-war activities, George Ohsawa and his associates formed the Centre Ignoramus, also called World Government Association, in Hiyoshi, a town between Tokyo and Yokohama, There, during a period from 1946 to 1952, the unifying principle,yin and yang, based upon the understanding of the order of the universe, was taught to young people of the postwar society. In 1952, the Center was moved to Yoyogi, Tokyo. Soon after that, George and Lima Ohsawa started on their world tour, spending time to stay and teach people in India and Africa. After they had the experience of living with Dr. Albert Schweitzer in Lambarene, Africa, they traveled to France and Belgium, and visited a few other European countries to spread macrobiotics—the application of the unifying principle to the problem of health. As a result of their influence, the macrobiotic movement began in these European countries, including food production and distribution.

Before that time, in 1949, Michio Kushi, during his postgraduate studies at Tokyo University, was inspired by the teaching of George Ohsawa. He came to the United States in connection with the World Federalist movement. Besides him, Aveline Tomoko Yokoyama in 1951, Herman Aihara in 1953, Cornellia Chiko Yokota, Romain Noboru Sato and his brothers Junsei Yamazaki, Shizuko Yamamoto, Noboru Muramoto and others came to the United States during the following years. After experience with various enterprises they respectively began to teach macrobiotics, mainly in New York. George and Lima Ohsawa also visited America from Europe to conduct seminars. Macrobiotic summer camps, restaurants, and food stores began to operate on a small scale with many American people. Educational activity was organized as the Ohsawa Foundation at that time. However, on the occasion of the Berlin Crisis in 1961, the major active people related to the macrobiotic movement made an "exodus" to Chico, California. Robert Kennedy, Lou Oles, Herman Aihara and others began Chico San, Inc., as a food manufacturing and distributing company, and established the Ohsawa Foundation in California. Later, the Foundation moved to Los Angeles, its main activity being publishing George Ohsawa's works. The San Francisco center was established. At a later date, Jacques and Yvette de Langre, Joe and Mimi Arseguel and many others shared educational activities in California and other areas of the West Coast.

In the meantime, after educational activity in New York, besides several seminars on Martha's Vineyard and various local colleges, Michio and Aveline Kushi moved to Boston in order to concentrate on education for the younger generations.They organized the East West Institute in Cambridge which later moved to Wellesley and then transferred to Boston. To meet the increasing demand for good food, a small basement food store, Erewhon, was opened. Erewhon was managed and developed over the years by the Kushis, Evan Root, William Tara, Roger Hillyard and Paul Hawken. Erewhon was followed by a small restaurant, Sanae, managed at different times by Evan Root, Tyler Smith, and Richard Sandler. Lectures by Michio Kushi continued for five years in Arlington Street Church, Boston, with repeated visits to many major U.S. cities. Erewhon developed into a larger store, on Newbury Street in Boston, and added its wholesale operation from a warehouse on the South Shore, Boston Wharf, distributing constantly to an increasing number of natural food stores. The warehouse facility has been managed by Paul Hawken, William Garrison, Tyler Smith, and currently Jeff Flasher and other associates as well as the Kushis. Erewhon further established a Los Angeles store which also developed into a wholesale operation—managed over the years by the Kushis, William Tara, Bruce MacDonald, and currently by John Fountain and Thomas DeSilva.

To meet the demands of increasing business, Sanae Restaurant opened an additional larger restaurant, the Seventh Inn, which has been managed by the Kushis, Yuko Okada, and currently by Hiroshi Hayashi. The examples of both Erewhon and the Seventh Inn have been followed by many new natural food stores and restaurants—such as Sanae West in Los Angeles, managed by Caroline Heidenry and associates—throughout the United States and Canada, many of which were established and are being operated by people who have studied in Boston. Up to 1977, more than ten distributors of high-quality natural foods have been in operation, covering nearly 10,000 retailers and co-operatives, and more than 300 natural food restaurants are in operation throughout North America. Though many of them are not directly managed according to the macrobiotic principles, it is obvious that they are serving for the betterment of the health of the general public.

In the meantime, the *East West Journal*, a monthly newspaper, established in 1970 —managed over the years by Ronald Dobrin, Jack Garvey, Robert Hargrove, and currently Sherman Goldman, Lenny Jacobs and other associates—is continuing to introduce to the wider society, the new vision for the present and future world. Educational activities directly concerned with teaching and other educational projects have been administered since 1973 by the East West Foundation, a nonprofit educational organization managed by the Kushis, Edward Esko, Stephen Uprichard, and other associates. Through the East West Foundation, many qualified assistant teachers have been participating in educational activities for the society at large. East West Centers have opened in many major cities in North America and since 1976, the Foundation expanded its state activities in Pennsylvania, Maryland, Washington D.C. and Florida, in coordination with the East West Centers. The Foundation, besides its regular educational programs including lectures, seminars, and publishing in Boston, is presenting classes in connection with several colleges and universities, either by arranging courses or by conducting seminars. The Foundation is also conducting the Ashburnham Land Project on 550 acres near Ashburnham, Mass., which is planned to be a comprehensive agricultural, educational and spiritual community based on the macrobiotic way of life. Construction and farming activities are in progress. The project is being administered by Woodward Johnson, Kimball Hart, and associates, as well the Kushis, with the special guidance of Mr. Granville Rideout.

In the Boston vicinity, several study houses were opened for the convenience of the people who come from other states and abroad. These study houses have been operated to offer experience in the macrobiotic way of life, teaching philosophy and practical applications in daily life. Senior house managers have been guiding the students, and out of the study houses many people return to their own cities and countries to inspire others. Currently among those seniors who are conducting study houses are Michael and Gretchen Swain, Kenneth and Ann Burns with Rod House, Jack and Barbara Garvey, Kit and Rob Allenson, Anita and Paul Miksis, Greg and Mutsuko Johnson, William and Andrea Kaufman, as far as the Boston vicinity is concerned. Educational activities cover not only the study of the order of the universe, but as its applications for health and well-being, include many aspects of the way of life and culture, including shiatsu massage, palm healing, acupuncture, moxibustion, yoga, Tai Chi Chuan, *Okido* exercise, tea ceremony, flower arrangement, and calligraphy as well as cooking, natural birth, natural farming—along with the spirit of respect and love for parents, ancestors and all people in society.

Through all the above activities, it is currently estimated that at least several million people in North America have turned to proper dietary practices using better quality of natural food, moving toward a healthy way of life. To meet the modern biological and psychological crisis, the East West Foundation, *East West Journal*, and other related activities have been focusing on solving the problems of cancer and other degenerative diseases since 1974. During this period medical seminars have been presented also, to more than 1,000 medical professionals, and occasionally special medical conferences have been held. The Foundation also publishes periodicals—"The Order of the Universe Magazine," "Kushi Seminar Reports," "Case History Report," "The Dietary Approach to Cancer," and many other reports.

In the meantime, natural organic farming has been spreading with the initiative of those who have been practicing the macrobiotic way of life. Those products, grown without the use of any chemical fertilizer or sprays, are supplied to local natural food distributors and stores. Natural quality cereal grains, beans, vegetables, and their products are constantly increasing in the market, including conventional supermarkets. *Tofu* and other soybean products, whole grain pasta and other whole cereal products have appeared during the past five years. *Miso, tamari* soy sauce, various seaweeds, and other high-quality foods are being imported from Japan and other countries, as supplements. Many books relating to the macrobiotic way of cooking and general way of health are being widely circulated. Among them are *You Are All Sanpaku* and *Sugar Blues* by William Dufty; *Cooking for Life* by Michel Abehsera; *The Art of Just Cooking* by Lima Ohsawa; and a series by the George Ohsawa Macrobiotic Foundation. Gloria Swanson, Jean Kohler, and many other people are also inspiring the general public.

Thus, a preliminary foundation has been laid for the betterment of the health of the people of North America. Kushi International Seminars have begun to be offered in European countries, covering many major cities with the cooperation of existing macrobiotic and Oriental culture establishments. The European Union for educational activities and the various centers of each country are influencing hundreds of thousands of people in Europe. Active education and good-quality food production and distribution are developing in all countries. The principle and practice of Oriental medicine have been introduced also through Kushi International Seminars and the educational activities of various centers, to establish the biological and psychological foundation for One Peaceful World.

Meanwhile, in 1975 the South Vietnamese Government opened a public macrobiotic restaurant in Saigon. In Central and South America since 1954 with the initiative of Tomio Kikuchi, Mr. Zanata and many other macrobiotic people, the way of life has been spreading, starting from Brazil. Besides Brazil, Venezuela, Argentina, Colombia, Uruguay, Mexico, and Costa Rica have many people who are practicing the macrobiotic way of life. In South Africa, the macrobiotic movement has been growing since 1974, and in Australia, very actively since 1976, initiated by Bruce Gingell and friends who studied in Boston. In the Soviet Union the interest in the macrobiotic way of life has been gradually growing for the past several years.

In Japan, the Nippon C.I. (Centre Ignoramus) in Tokyo, and Sekai Seishoku Kyokai (World Macrobiotic Organization) in Osaka have been initiating education together with macrobiotic centers in Kyoto, Nagoya, Hiroshima, and many other cities and provinces. They are each publishing books and periodicals as well as conducting lectures and seminars to develop consultants and to secure public health, preventing environment and food from contamination by the recent developments of industry.

As a whole, educational activities throughout the world are aiming to secure the biological and psychological health of mankind, to develop the quality of the human species through the proper understanding of natural law and the order of the universe, to synthesize Eastern and Western culture, philosophy and science, and to achieve One Peaceful World with the health, love, peace, and freedom of everyone in the world.

Composition of Foods, 100 grams, Edible Portion

(Numbers in parentheses denote values imputed—usually from another form of the food or from a similar food. Zero in parentheses indicates that the amount of a constituent probably is none or is too small to measure. Dashes denote lack of reliable data for a constituent believed to be present in measurable amount. Asterisk (*) indicates information unavailable. Calculated values, as those based on a recipe, are not in parentheses.) (Sources: U.S. Department of Agriculture and Japan Nutritionist Association)

Food and Description	Water	Food energy	Protein	Fat	Carbohydrates Total	Fiber	Ash	Calcium	Phosphorous	Iron	Sodium	Potassium	Vit. A	Vit. B₁ (Thiamin)	Vit. B₂ (Riboflavin)	Niacin (Nicotinic Acid)	Vit. C (Ascorbic Acid)
	%	Cal.	Grams	Grams	Grams	Grams	Grams	Mg.	Mg.	Mg.	Mg.	Mg.	I.U.	Mg.	Mg.	Mg.	Mg.
1. GRAINS																	
Barley (Pearled)	11.1	349	8.2	1.0	78.8	0.5	0.9	16	189	2.0	3	160	(0)	0.12	0.05	3.1	(0)
Buckwheat, whole grain	11.0	335	11.7	2.4	72.9	9.9	2.0	114	282	3.1	—	448	(0)	0.6	—	4.4	(0)
Corn, white and yellow	72.7	96	3.5	1.0	22.1	0.7	0.7	3	111	0.7	Trace	280	400	0.15	0.12	1.7	12
Cornmeal	12.0	355	9.2	3.9	73.7	1.6	1.2	20	256	2.4	(1)	(284)	510	0.38	0.11	2.0	(0)
Millet, whole grain	11.8	327	9.9	2.9	72.9	3.2	2.5	20	311	6.8	—	430	(0)	0.73	0.38	2.3	(0)
Noodles:																	
Soba (Dried)	13.5	360	10.8	1.8	73.0	0.4	0.9	30	210	5.0	700	*	0	0.20	0.08	1.2	0
Somen	14.0	341	8.4	1.3	71.8	0.3	4.5	24	110	1.8	1,200	*	0	0.12	0.04	1.0	0
Udon	72.0	116	2.6	0.3	24.9	0.1	0.2	5	25	0.3	120	*	0	0.04	0.01	0.2	0
Oats, whole grain	12.5	313	13.0	5.4	66.1	10.6	3.0	55	320	4.6	10	*	0	0.30	0.10	1.5	0
Oatmeal or rolled oats (Dried form)	8.3	390	14.2	7.4	68.2	1.2	1.9	53	405	4.5	2	352	(0)	0.60	0.14	1.0	(0)
Rice, brown, whole grain	12.0	360	7.5	1.9	77.4	0.9	1.2	32	221	1.6	9	214	(0)	0.34	0.05	4.7	(0)
Brown rice *mochi*	15.5	336	7.6	2.3	73.2	1.2	1.4	10	290	1.1	3	*	0	0.36	0.10	4.5	(0)
Rice, white	15.5	351	6.2	0.8	76.9	0.3	0.6	6	150	0.4	2	*	0	0.09	0.03	1.4	0
White rice *mochi*	40.0	249	4.5	0.4	54.8	0.3	0.3	4	60	0.3	2	*	0	0.04	0.02	1.0	0
Rye, whole grain	11.0	357	9.4	1.0	77.9	0.4	0.7	22	185	1.1	(1)	156	(0)	0.15	0.07	0.6	(0)
Wheat, whole grain (Hard, red spring)	13.0	330	14.0	2.2	69.1	2.3	1.7	36	383	3.1	(3)	370	(0)	0.59	0.12	4.3	(0)
Wheat flour (Whole, from hard wheat)	12.0	333	13.3	2.0	71.0	2.3	1.7	41	372	3.3	3	370	(0)	0.55	0.12	4.3	(0)
2. BEANS (Uncooked)																	
Azuki	15.5	326	21.5	1.6	58.4	4.3	3.0	75	350	4.8	7	*	6	0.50	0.10	2.5	0

Chickpeas (Garbanzos)	10.7	360	20.5	4.8	61.0	5.0	3.0	150	331	6.9	26	797	50	0.31	0.15	2.0	—
Lentils, whole	11.1	340	24.7	1.1	60.1	3.9	3.0	79	377	6.8	30	790	60	0.37	0.22	2.0	—
Mung beans, sprouted	88.8	35	3.8	0.2	6.6	0.7	0.6	19	64	1.3	5	223	20	0.13	0.13	0.8	19
Dried Peas	11.7	340	24.1	1.3	60.3	4.9	2.6	64	340	5.1	35	1,005	120	0.74	0.29	3.0	—
Pinto, calico, and Mexican	8.3	349	22.9	1.2	63.7	4.3	3.9	135	457	6.4	10	984	—	0.84	0.21	2.2	—
Soybeans, raw	10.0	403	34.1	17.7	33.5	4.9	4.7	226	554	8.4	5	1,677	80	1.10	0.31	2.2	—
Natto (Fermented soybeans)	62.7	167	16.9	7.4	11.5	3.2	1.5	103	182	3.7	—	249	0	0.07	0.50	1.1	0
Miso:																	
Hacho	47.5	180	16.8	6.9	15.8	2.2	13.0	140	240	6.5	3,800	*	0	0.04	0.12	1.2	0
Mugi (Barley and soybeans)	50.0	156	14.0	5.0	16.2	1.9	14.8	115	190	4.0	4,600	*	0	0.03	0.10	1.5	0
Soybean curd (*Tofu*)	84.8	72	7.8	4.2	2.4	0.1	0.8	128	126	1.9	7	42	0	0.06	0.03	0.1	0
Okara	84.5	65	3.5	1.9	9.2	2.3	0.9	76	43	1.4	4	*	0	0.07	0.56	1.1	0
Soybean sprouts	86.3	46	6.2	1.4	5.3	0.8	0.8	48	67	1.0	—	—	80	0.23	0.20	0.8	13
3. POTATO and STARCHES																	
Corn Starch	92.8	21	2.0	0.4	3.6	0.8	1.2	—	—	—	7	*	—	—	—	—	—
Jinenjo	68.0	121	3.5	0.1	27.5	0.9	0.9	21	46	0.7	2	*	0	0.08	0.02	1.0	5
Kuzu	16.5	336	0.2	0.1	83.1	0	0.1	17	10	2.0	3	*	0	0.10	0	1.5	0
Potato, white	79.8	76	2.1	0.1	17.1	0.5	0.9	7	53	0.6	10	407	Trace	0.10	0.04	0.6	20
Sweet Potato	70.6	114	1.7	0.4	26.3	0.7	1.0	32	47	0.7	7	243	8,800	0.13	0.06	1.1	21
Taro Potato	73.0	98	1.9	0.2	23.7	0.8	1.2	28	61	1.0	—	514	20	—	0.04	—	4
4. SUGAR and SWEETENERS																	
Chocolate Syrup	31.6	245	2.3	2.0	62.7	0.6	1.0	17	92	1.6	52	282	Trace	0.02	0.07	0.4	0
Honey	17.2	304	0.3	0	82.3	—	0.2	5	6	0.5	5	51	0	Trace	0.04	0.3	1
Maple Syrup	8.0	348	—	—	90.0	—	0.9	143	11	1.4	14	242	—	—	—	—	0
Mizu-ame (Rice starch sweetener)	17.0	321	0	0	83.0	0	0	2	1	0.1	1	*	0	0	0	0	0
Molasses	24.0	232	—	—	60.0	—	8.5	290	69	6.0	37	1,063	—	—	0.12	1.2	—
Raw Sugar (brown)	2.1	373	0	0	96.4	0	1.5	85	19	3.4	30	344	0	0.01	0.03	0.2	0
White Sugar	0.5	385	0	0	99.5	0	Trace	0	0	0.1	1	3	0	0	0	0	0
5. OIL and FATS																	
Butter	15.5	716	0.6	81.0	0.4	0	2.5	20	16	0	987	23	3,300	—	—	0	0
Lard	0	902	0	100	0	0	0	0	0	0	0	0	0	0	0	—	0
Margarine	15.5	720	0.6	81.0	0.4	0	2.5	20	16	0	987	23	3,300	—	—	0	0
Vegetable oil	0	884	0	100	0	0	0	0	0	0	0	0	0	0	0	—	0
6. SEEDS and NUTS																	
Almonds	4.7	598	18.6	54.2	19.5	2.6	3.0	234	504	4.7	4	773	0	0.24	0.92	3.5	Trace

Food and Description	Water %	Food energy Cal.	Protein Grams	Fat Grams	Carbohydrates Total Grams	Fiber Grams	Ash Grams	Calcium Mg.	Phosphorous Mg.	Iron Mg.	Sodium Mg.	Potassium Mg.	Vit. A I.U.	Vit. B₁ (Thiamin) Mg.	Vit. B₂ (Riboflavin) Mg.	Niacin (Nicotinic Acid) Mg.	Vit. C (Ascorbic Acid) Mg.
Brazil nuts	4.6	654	14.3	66.9	10.9	3.1	3.3	186	693	3.4	1	715	Trace	0.96	0.12	1.6	—
Cashews	5.2	561	17.2	45.7	29.3	1.4	2.6	38	373	3.8	15	464	100	0.43	0.25	1.8	—
Chestnuts (fresh)	52.5	194	2.9	1.5	42.1	1.1	1.0	27	88	1.7	6	454	—	0.22	0.22	0.6	—
Filberts (hazelnuts)	5.8	634	12.6	62.4	16.7	3.0	2.5	209	337	3.4	2	704	—	0.46	—	0.9	Trace
Peanuts	5.6	564	26.0	47.5	18.6	2.4	2.3	69	401	2.1	5	674	—	1.14	0.13	17.2	0
Peanut Butter	1.8	581	27.8	49.4	17.2	1.9	3.8	63	407	2.0	607	670	—	0.13	0.13	15.7	0
Pecans	3.4	687	9.2	71.2	14.6	2.3	1.6	73	289	2.4	Trace	603	130	0.86	0.13	0.9	2
Pine nuts	5.6	552	31.1	47.4	11.6	0.9	4.3	—	—	—	—	—	—	0.62	—	—	—
Pumpkin Seeds	4.4	553	29.0	46.7	15.0	1.9	4.9	51	1,144	11.2	—	—	70	0.24	0.19	2.4	—
Sesame Seeds	5.4	563	18.6	49.1	21.6	6.3	5.3	1,160	616	10.5	60	725	30	0.98	0.24	5.4	0
Sunflower Seeds	4.8	560	24.0	47.3	19.9	3.8	4.0	120	837	7.1	30	920	50	1.96	0.23	5.4	—
Walnuts (English)	3.5	651	14.8	64.0	15.8	2.1	1.9	99	380	3.1	2	450	30	0.33	0.13	0.9	2

7. FISH and SHELLFISH

FISH:

Food and Description	Water %	Food energy Cal.	Protein Grams	Fat Grams	Carbohydrates Total Grams	Fiber Grams	Ash Grams	Calcium Mg.	Phosphorous Mg.	Iron Mg.	Sodium Mg.	Potassium Mg.	Vit. A I.U.	Vit. B₁ Mg.	Vit. B₂ Mg.	Niacin Mg.	Vit. C Mg.
Bass, striped	77.7	105	18.9	2.7	0	0	1.2	—	212	—	—	—	—	—	—	—	—
Bluefish	75.4	117	20.5	5.3	0	0	1.2	23	243	0.6	74	—	—	0.12	0.09	1.9	—
Bonita	67.6	168	24.0	7.3	0	0	1.4	—	—	—	—	—	—	—	—	—	—
Carp	77.8	115	18.0	4.2	0	0	1.1	50	253	0.9	50	286	170	0.01	0.04	1.5	1
Codfish	81.2	78	17.6	0.3	0	0	1.2	10	194	0.4	70	382	0	0.06	0.07	2.2	2
Eel	64.6	233	15.9	18.3	0	0	1.0	18	202	0.7	—	—	1,610	0.22	0.36	1.4	—
Flatfishes (Flounders, soles, and sanddabs)	81.3	79	16.7	0.8	0	0	1.2	12	195	0.8	78	342	—	0.05	0.05	1.7	—
Haddock	80.5	79	18.3	0.1	0	0	1.4	23	197	0.7	61	304	—	0.04	0.07	3.0	—
Herring	69.0	176	17.3	11.3	0	0	2.1	—	256	1.1	—	—	110	0.02	0.15	3.6	—
Mackerel	67.2	191	19.0	12.2	0	0	1.6	5	239	1.0	—	—	(450)	0.15	0.33	8.2	—
Salmon	63.6	217	22.5	13.4	0	0	1.4	79	186	0.9	—	—	220	—	0.08	7.2	9
Sardine	61.8	203	24.0	11.1	—	—	3.1	437	499	2.9	823	590	220	0.03	0.20	5.4	—
Smelt	79.0	98	18.6	2.1	0	0	1.1	—	272	0.4	—	—	—	0.01	0.12	1.4	—
Snapper	78.5	93	19.8	0.9	0	0	1.3	16	214	0.8	67	323	—	0.17	0.02	—	—
Trout, rainbow	66.3	195	21.5	11.4	0	0	1.3	—	—	—	—	—	—	0.08	0.20	8.4	—
Tuna	70.5	145	25.2	4.1	0	0	1.3	—	—	1.3	—	—	—	—	—	—	—
Whitefish, lake	71.7	155	18.9	8.2	0	0	1.2	—	270	0.4	52	299	2,260	0.14	0.12	3.0	—

SHELLFISH:

Food and Description	Water %	Food energy Cal.	Protein Grams	Fat Grams	Carbohydrates Total Grams	Fiber Grams	Ash Grams	Calcium Mg.	Phosphorous Mg.	Iron Mg.	Sodium Mg.	Potassium Mg.	Vit. A I.U.	Vit. B₁ Mg.	Vit. B₂ Mg.	Niacin Mg.	Vit. C Mg.
Abalone	75.8	98	18.7	0.5	3.4	0	1.6	37	191	2.4	—	—	—	0.18	0.14	—	—

Food																
Clams	85.8	54	8.6	1.0	2.0	—	2.6	—	208	—	—	—	—	—	—	—	—
Shortnecked clam	85.4	63	10.6	1.3	1.5	0	1.2	80	180	7	200	*	180	0.04	0.15	1.5	10
King crab	78.5	93	17.3	1.9	0.5	—	1.8	43	175	0.8	—	—	2,170	0.16	0.08	2.8	2
Octopus	82.2	73	15.3	0.8	0	0	1.5	29	173	—	—	—	—	0.02	0.06	1.8	—
Oyster	84.6	66	8.4	1.8	3.4	—	1.8	94	143	5.5	73	121	310	0.14	0.18	2.5	—
Squid	80.2	84	16.4	0.9	1.5	—	1.0	12	119	0.5	—	—	—	0.02	0.12	—	—
8. MEAT and POULTRY																
Beef, sirloin	55.7	313	16.9	26.7	0	0	0.8	10	155	2.5	65	355	50	0.07	0.15	4.1	—
Hamburger—ground beef	60.2	268	17.9	21.2	0	0	0.7	10	156	2.7	—	236	40	0.08	0.16	4.3	0
Bullfrog	78.8	88	19.9	0.3	0	0	1.0	3	140	0.3	—	*	15	0.10	0.06	1.2	1
Chicken	63.0	239	18.2	17.9	0	0	0.9	10	176	1.6	—	—	920	0.08	0.19	6.7	—
Duck	54.3	326	16.0	28.6	0	0	1.0	(10)	(176)	(1.6)	—	—	—	(0.08)	(0.19)	(6.7)	—
EGGS:																
Duck eggs	70.4	191	13.3	14.5	0.7	0	1.1	56	195	2.8	(122)	(129)	1,230	0.18	(0.30)	0.1	0
Chicken eggs (Whole)	73.7	163	12.9	11.5	0.9	0	1.0	54	205	2.3	122	129	1,180	0.11	0.30	0.1	0
(Yolk)	51.1	348	16.0	30.6	0.6	0	0.7	9	15	0.1	146	139	0	Trace	0.27	0.1	0
(White)	87.6	51	10.9	Trace	0.8	0	0.7	9	15	0.1	146	139	0	Trace	0.27	0.1	0
Goat Meat	74.2	123	20.6	3.8	0.1	0	1.3	8	—	2	90	*	0	0.15	0.08	4.0	0
Horsemeat	73.6	125	20.5	3.7	1.0	0	1.2	4	200	2	100	*	20	0.10	0.10	3.5	0
Lamb	60.8	262	16.9	21.0	0	0	1.3	10	152	1.3	75	295	—	0.15	0.21	4.9	0
Pheasant	69.2	151	24.3	5.2	0	0	1.2	—	—	—	—	—	—	—	—	—	—
9. DAIRY FOOD																
CHEESE:																
Cheddar (American)	37.0	398	25.0	32.2	2.1	0	3.7	750	478	1.0	700	82	(1,310)	0.03	0.46	0.1	(0)
Cottage	78.3	106	13.6	4.2	2.9	0	1.0	94	152	0.3	229	85	(170)	0.03	0.25	0.1	(0)
Edam	33.8	389	31.7	28.4	1.0	0	5.1	850	640	0.6	1,300	*	1,100	0.04	0.50	0.3	0
Cream, raw	71.5	211	3.0	20.6	4.3	0	0.6	102	80	Trace	43	122	840	0.03	0.15	0.1	1
Ice Cream	63.2	193	4.5	10.6	20.8	0	0.9	146	115	0.1	63	181	440	0.04	0.21	0.1	1
MILK:																
Condensed Milk	27.1	321	8.1	8.7	54.3	0	1.8	262	206	0.1	112	314	360	0.08	0.38	0.2	1
Dry Milk (Powder)	2.0	502	26.4	27.5	38.2	0	5.9	909	708	0.5	405	1,330	1,130	0.29	1.46	0.7	6
Goat's Milk	87.5	67	3.2	4.0	4.6	0	0.7	129	106	0.1	34	180	(160)	0.04	0.11	0.3	1
Human Milk	88.2	61	1.4	3.1	7.1	0	0.2	35	25	0.2	15	*	120	0.02	0.03	0.2	5
Skim Milk	90.5	36	3.6	1	5.1	0	0.7	121	95	Trace	52	145	Trace	0.04	0.18	0.1	1
Whole Milk	87.4	65	3.5	3.5	4.9	0	0.7	118	93	Trace	50	144	140	0.03	0.17	0.1	1
Sherbet	67.0	134	0.9	1.2	30.8	0	0.1	16	13	Trace	10	22	60	0.01	0.03	Trace	2
Yogurt	89.0	50	3.4	1.7	5.2	0	0.7	120	94	Trace	51	143	74	0.04	0.18	0.1	1
10. VEGETABLES (Uncooked)																
Asparagus	91.7	26	2.5	0.2	5.0	0.7	0.6	22	62	1.0	2	278	900	0.18	0.20	1.5	33
Bamboo Shoot	91.0	27	2.6	0.3	5.2	0.7	0.9	13	59	0.5	—	533	20	0.15	0.07	0.6	4

Food and Description	Water %	Food energy Cal.	Protein Grams	Fat Grams	Carbohydrates Total Grams	Fiber Grams	Ash Grams	Calcium Mg.	Phosphorous Mg.	Iron Mg.	Sodium Mg.	Potassium Mg.	Vit. A I.U.	Vit. B₁ (Thiamin) Mg.	Vit. B₂ (Riboflavin) Mg.	Niacin (Nicotinic Acid) Mg.	Vit. C (Ascorbic Acid) Mg.
Beets	87.3	43	1.6	0.1	9.9	0.8	1.1	16	33	0.7	60	335	20	0.03	0.05	0.4	10
Beet greens	90.9	24	2.2	0.3	4.6	1.3	2.0	119	40	3.3	130	570	6,100	0.10	0.22	0.4	30
Broad Beans	72.3	105	8.4	0.4	17.8	2.2	1.1	27	157	2.2	4	471	220	0.28	0.17	1.6	30
Broccoli	89.1	32	3.6	0.3	5.9	1.5	1.1	103	78	1.1	15	382	2,500	0.10	0.23	0.9	113
Brussels Sprouts	85.2	45	4.9	0.4	8.3	1.6	1.2	36	80	1.5	14	390	550	0.10	0.16	0.9	102
Burdock	78.8	75	4.1	0.1	16.3	1.5	0.7	47	71	0.8	45	*	0	0.30	0.05	0	2
Cabbage, common	92.4	24	1.3	0.2	5.4	0.8	0.7	49	29	0.4	20	233	130	0.05	0.05	0.3	47
Cabbage, Chinese	95.0	14	1.2	0.1	3.0	0.6	0.7	43	40	0.6	23	253	150	0.05	0.04	0.6	25
Carrots	83.2	42	1.1	0.2	9.7	1.0	0.8	37	36	0.7	47	341	11,000	0.06	0.05	0.6	8
Cauliflower	91.0	27	2.7	0.2	5.2	1.0	0.9	25	56	1.1	13	295	60	0.11	0.10	0.7	78
Celery	94.1	17	0.9	0.1	3.9	0.6	1.0	39	28	0.3	126	341	240	0.03	0.03	0.3	9
Collard Greens	86.9	40	3.6	0.7	7.2	0.9	1.6	203	63	1.0	43	401	6,500	0.20	(0.31)	(1.7)	92
Cucumber	95.1	15	0.9	0.1	3.4	0.6	0.5	25	27	1.1	6	160	250	0.03	0.04	0.2	11
Daikon (Long radish)	94.1	19	0.9	0.1	4.2	0.7	0.7	35	26	0.6	—	180	10	0.03	0.02	0.4	32
Daikon Leaves	83.5	49	5.2	0.7	8.5	1.4	2.1	190	30	1.4	100	*	3,000	0.10	0.30	0.5	90
Dandelion Greens	85.6	45	2.7	0.7	9.2	1.6	1.8	187	66	3.1	76	397	14,000	0.19	0.26	—	35
Eggplant	92.4	25	1.2	0.2	5.6	0.9	0.6	12	26	0.7	2	214	10	0.05	0.05	0.6	5
Garlic	61.3	137	6.2	0.2	30.8	1.5	1.5	29	202	1.5	1.9	529	Trace	0.25	0.08	0.5	15
Ginger root, fresh	87.0	49	1.4	1.0	9.5	1.1	1.1	23	36	2.1	6	264	10	0.20	0.04	0.7	4
Green peas	78.0	84	6.3	0.4	14.4	2.0	0.9	26	116	1.9	2	316	640	0.35	0.14	2.9	27
Kale	87.5	38	4.2	0.8	6.0	1.3	1.5	179	73	2.2	75	378	8,900	—	—	—	125
Lettuce (Iceberg)	95.5	13	0.9	0.1	2.9	0.5	0.6	20	22	0.5	9	175	330	0.06	0.06	0.3	6
Lotus	82.6	62	2.4	0.1	14.3	0.9	0.6	20	80	0.5	30	*	0	0.05	0.03	0.5	20
Mushrooms:																	
Common varieties	90.4	28	2.7	0.3	4.4	0.8	0.9	6	116	0.8	15	414	Trace	0.10	0.46	4.2	3
Shiitake	15.8	—	12.5	1.6	65.5	5.5	4.6	16	240	0.39	—	*	0	0.32	0.74	10.0	0
Mustard greens	89.5	31	3.0	0.5	5.6	1.1	1.4	183	50	3.0	32	377	7,000	0.11	0.22	0.8	97
Okra	88.9	36	2.4	0.3	7.6	1.0	0.8	92	51	0.6	3	249	520	(0.17)	(0.21)	(1.0)	31
Onions	89.1	38	1.5	0.1	8.7	0.6	0.6	27	36	0.5	10	157	40	0.03	0.04	0.2	10
Parsley	85.1	44	3.6	0.6	8.5	1.5	2.2	203	63	6.2	45	727	8,500	0.12	0.26	1.2	172
Parsnips	79.1	76	1.7	0.5	17.5	2.0	1.2	50	77	0.7	12	541	30	0.08	0.09	0.2	16
Peppers:																	
Red	74.3	93	3.7	2.3	18.1	9.0	1.6	29	78	1.2	—	—	21,600	0.22	0.36	4.4	369
Sweet	93.4	22	1.2	0.2	4.8	1.4	0.4	9	22	0.7	13	213	420	0.08	0.08	0.5	128
Pumpkin	91.6	26	1.0	0.1	6.5	1.1	0.8	21	44	0.8	1	340	1,600	0.05	0.11	0.6	9

Scallion	89.4	36	1.5	0.2	8.2	(1.2)	0.7	51	39	1.0	5	231	(2,000)	0.05	0.05	0.4	32
Spinach	90.7	26	3.2	0.3	4.3	0.6	1.5	93	51	3.1	71	470	8,100	0.10	0.20	0.6	51
Squash:																	
Summer	94.0	19	1.1	0.1	4.2	0.6	0.6	28	29	0.4	1	202	410	0.05	0.09	1.0	22
Winter	85.1	50	1.4	0.3	12.4	1.4	0.8	22	38	0.6	1	369	3,700	0.05	0.11	0.6	13
Swiss Chard	91.1	25	2.4	0.3	4.6	0.8	1.6	88	39	3.2	147	550	6,500	0.06	0.17	0.5	32
Tomato	93.5	22	1.1	0.2	4.7	0.5	0.5	13	27	0.5	3	244	900	0.06	0.04	0.7	23
Wild Grass:																	
Bracken, fresh	88.6	36	2.3	0.4	7.5	1.0	1.2	11	19	1.1	—	*	66	0	0.30	3.5	30
Bracken, dried	13.0	253	26.8	1.2	49.6	12.6	9.4	75	100	8.0	—	*	660	0	0.30	4.2	0
Royal Fern, fresh	88.3	38	3.1	0.2	8.1	3.8	0.3	9	18	0.8	—	*	16	0	0.40	0.7	15
Royal Fern, dried	19.9	257	17.6	2.7	53.7	8.4	6.1	65	100	6.0	—	*	0	0	0.40	1.2	0
Horsetail	93.7	20	1.0	0.2	4.4	1.1	0.7	58	93	4.4	—	*	500	0	0.07	5.6	50
Japanese Mugwort	87.2	35	5.2	0.8	4.5	3.0	2.3	70	25	1.5	—	*	2,300	0.15	0.28	3.0	70
New Zealand Spinach	93.8	15	2.1	0.3	2.1	0.5	1.7	48	77	3.0	—	*	1,800	0.08	0.30	1.0	40
Shepherd's Purse	86.4	39	4.5	0.5	6.6	1.1	2.0	300	94	2.5	—	*	830	0.16	0.28	0.5	40
11. FRUITS																	
Apples	84.4	58	0.2	0.6	14.5	1.0	0.3	7	10	0.3	1	110	90	0.03	0.02	0.1	4
Apple juice	87.8	47	0.1	Trace	11.9	0.1	0.2	6	9	0.6	1	101	—	0.01	0.02	0.1	1
Apricot	85.3	51	1.0	0.2	12.8	0.6	0.7	17	23	0.5	1	281	2,700	0.03	0.04	0.6	10
Avocado	74.0	167	2.1	16.4	6.3	1.6	1.2	10	42	0.6	4	604	290	0.11	0.20	1.6	14
Banana	75.7	85	1.1	0.2	22.2	0.5	0.8	8	26	0.7	1	370	190	0.05	0.06	0.7	10
Cherries	80.4	70	1.3	0.3	17.4	0.4	0.6	22	19	0.4	2	191	110	0.05	0.06	0.4	10
Dates	22.5	274	2.2	0.5	72.9	2.3	1.9	59	63	3.0	1	648	50	0.09	0.10	2.2	0
Figs	77.5	80	1.2	0.3	20.3	1.2	0.7	35	22	0.6	2	194	80	0.06	0.05	0.4	2
Grapefruit	84.4	41	0.5	0.1	10.6	0.2	0.4	16	16	0.4	1	135	80	0.04	0.02	0.2	38
Grapes	81.6	69	1.3	1.0	15.7	0.6	0.4	16	12	0.4	3	158	100	(0.05)	(0.03)	(0.3)	4
Kumquat	81.3	65	0.9	0.1	17.1	3.7	0.6	63	23	0.4	7	236	600	0.08	0.10	—	36
Lemon	87.4	20	1.2	0.3	10.7	—	0.4	61	15	0.7	3	145	30	0.05	0.04	0.2	77
Nectarine	81.8	64	0.6	Trace	17.1	0.4	0.5	4	24	0.5	6	294	1,650	—	—	—	13
Orange	86.0	49	1.0	0.2	12.2	0.5	0.6	41	20	0.4	1	200	200	0.10	0.04	0.4	(50)
Orange juice	88.3	45	0.7	0.2	10.4	0.1	0.4	11	17	0.2	1	200	200	0.09	0.03	0.4	50
Papaya	88.7	39	0.6	0.1	10.0	0.9	0.6	20	16	0.3	3	234	1,750	0.04	0.04	0.3	56
Peaches	89.1	38	0.6	0.1	9.7	0.6	0.5	9	19	0.5	1	202	1,330	0.02	0.05	1.0	7
Pears	83.2	61	0.7	0.4	15.3	1.4	0.4	8	11	0.3	2	130	20	0.02	0.04	0.1	4
Persimmon	64.4	127	0.8	0.4	33.5	1.5	0.9	27	26	2.5	1	310	—	—	—	—	66
Pineapple	85.3	52	0.4	0.2	13.7	0.4	0.4	17	8	0.5	1	146	70	0.09	0.03	0.2	17
Plum	81.1	66	0.5	Trace	17.8	0.4	0.6	18	17	0.5	2	299	(300)	0.08	0.03	0.5	—
Raisins	18.0	289	2.5	0.2	77.4	0.9	1.9	62	101	3.5	27	763	20	0.11	0.08	0.5	1
Strawberries	89.9	37	0.7	0.5	8.4	1.3	0.5	21	21	1.0	1	164	60	0.03	0.07	0.6	59
Tangerines	87	46	0.8	0.2	11.6	0.5	0.4	40	18	0.4	2	126	420	0.06	0.02	0.1	31
Watermelon	92.6	26	0.5	0.2	6.4	0.3	0.3	7	10	0.5	1	100	590	0.03	0.03	0.2	7

Food and Description	Water	Food energy	Protein	Fat	Carbohydrates Total	Carbohydrates Fiber	Ash	Calcium	Phosphorous	Iron	Sodium	Potassium	Vit. A	Vit. B1 (Thiamin)	Vit. B2 (Riboflavin)	Niacin (Nicotinic Acid)	Vit. C (Ascorbic Acid)
	%	Cal.	Grams	Grams	Grams	Grams	Grams	Mg.	Mg.	Mg.	Mg.	Mg.	I.U.	Mg.	Mg.	Mg.	Mg.
12. SEAWEEDS																	
Agar-agar (Kanten)	20.1	—	2.3	0.1	74.6	0	2.9	400	8	5	—	*	0	0	0	0	0
Arame	19.3	—	7.5	0.1	60.6	9.8	12.5	1,170	150	12	—	*	50	0.02	0.20	2.6	0
Dulse	16.6	—	—	3.0	—	0.7	3.7	567	22	6.3	—	*	150	0.01	0.20	4.0	0
Hijiki	16.8	—	5.6	0.8	42.8	13.0	34.0	1,400	56	29	—	*	—	—	—	—	—
Kelp	21.7	—	—	1.1	—	6.8	22.8	1,093	240	—	3,007	5,273	—	—	—	—	—
Kombu	14.7	—	7.3	1.1	54.9	3.0	22.0	800	150	—	2,500	*	430	0.08	0.32	1.8	11
Nori	11.4	—	35.6	0.7	44.3	4.7	8.0	260	510	12	600	*	11,000	0.25	1.24	10.0	20
Wakame	16.0	—	12.7	1.5	51.4	3.6	18.4	1,300	260	13	2,500	*	140	0.11	0.14	10	15
13. BEVERAGES																	
Beer	92.1	42	0.3	0	3.8	—	0.2	5	30	Trace	7	25	—	Trace	0.03	0.6	—
Coffee	98.1	1	Trace	Trace	Trace	Trace	0.1	2	4	0.1	1	36	0	0	Trace	0.3	0
Gin, rum, vodka, whiskey:																	
80-proof	66.6	231	—	—	Trace	—	—	—	—	—	1	2	—	—	—	—	—
100-proof	57.5	295	—	—	Trace	—	—	—	—	—	1	2	—	—	—	—	—
Sake (Rice wine)	—	110	0.5	0	5.0	0	0	5	6	0.1	—	*	0	0	0	0	0
Tea:																	
Bancha (Twig Tea)	7.0	—	20.3	4.3	61.0	19.0	5.4	720	200	37.0	60	*	9,000	0.08	0.89	9.0	130
Black Tea	9.0	—	22.6	2.4	58.2	10.7	5.1	460	310	17.0	50	*	1,300	0.09	0.56	10.0	0
Green Tea	6.0	—	31.6	4.6	49.6	10.6	5.4	440	280	20.0	60	*	9,000	0.35	1.40	4.0	280
Wine:																	
Dessert (Alcohol 18.8% by volume)	76.7	137	0.1	0	7.7	—	0.2	8	—	—	4	75	—	0.01	0.02	0.2	—
Table (Alcohol 12.2% by volume)	85.6	85	0.1	0	4.2	—	0.2	9	10	0.4	5	92	—	Trace	0.01	0.1	—
14. SEASONING																	
Horseradish, prepared	87.1	38	1.3	0.2	9.6	0.9	1.8	61	32	0.9	96	290	—	—	—	—	—
Mayonnaise	15.1	718	1.1	79.9	2.2	Trace	1.7	18	28	0.5	597	34	280	0.02	0.04	Trace	0
Pepper	10.6	—	8.7	5.5	58.8	2.6	16.4	—	—	—	—	*	0	0	0	0	0
Tamari Soy Sauce	62.8	68	5.6	1.3	9.5	0	20.8	82	104	4.8	7,325	366	0	0.02	0.25	0.4	0
Tomato Catsup	68.6	106	2.0	0.4	25.4	0.5	3.6	22	50	0.8	1,042	363	1,400	0.09	0.07	1.6	15
Umeboshi	69.8	17	0.3	0.8	3.4	0.3	25.7	6.1	26	2.0	9,400	*	0	0.06	0.09	0.6	0
Vinegar	93.8	14	Trace	(0)	5.9	—	0.3	(6)	(9)	(0.6)	1	100	—	—	—	—	—
Takka-Miso	40.0	249	9.0	5.2	42.8	2.0	3.0	150	250	60	*	*	0	0.10	0.15	1.5	0

Educational and Cultural Activities

East West Foundations

Florida
East West Foundation
3921 S.W. 60th Court
Miami, Fla. 33155

Maryland
East West Foundation
6209 Park Heights Ave.
Baltimore, MD 21215

Massachusetts
East West Foundation
359 Boylston St.
Boston, Mass. 02116

Pennsylvania
East West Foundation
6 Radcliffe Rd.
Bala Cynwyd, Pa. 19004

Washington D.C.
East West Foundation
P.O. Box 40012
Washington, D.C. 20016

East West Center Affiliates

California
East West Center
P.O. Box 37
Forestville, CA 95436

East West Center
7511 Franklin Ave.
Hollywood, CA 90046

Vega Institute
P.O. Box 426
Oroville, CA 95965

East West Center
2731 Fleetwood Dr.
San Bruno, CA 94066

Colorado
East West Center
1013 Venus
Colorado Springs, Colo. 80906

Illinois
East West Center
2525 W. Gunnison St.
Chicago, Ill. 60625

Indiana
East West Center
2900 Torquay Rd.
Muncie. IN 47304

Massachusetts
East West Center
32 Burncoat St.
Worcester, Mass. 01605

Minnesota
East West Center
993 Portland Ave.
St. Paul, MN 55104

New York
East West Center
142 West 44th St.
New York, N.Y. 10023

Ohio
East West Center
347 Ludlow Ave.
Cincinnati. OH 45220

Washington
East West Center
264-A.E. Newton
Seattle, WA 98102

CANADA
East West Center
Box 1620
Fernie, B.C.

East West Center
696 W. 20th Ave.
Vancouver, B.C.

East West Center
10 Brook Ave.
Toronto, Ont.

ENGLAND
Community Health Foundation
East West Center
188 Old St.
London, ECI

Quality Food Restaurants

California
Good Karma Cafe
501 Dolores St.
San Francisco, Calif. 94110

Florida
Oak Feed Restaurant
3008 Grand Ave.
Coconut Grove, Fla. 33133

Su-shin Restaurant
3339 Virginia Ave.
Coconut Grove, Fla. 33133

Illinois
Plowshare Natural Food Restaurant
6155 N. Broadway
Chicago, Ill. 60660

Indiana
Harvest Moon Restaurant
207 North Bill St.
Muncie, Ind. 47303

Massachusetts
Sanae Restaurant
272A Newbury St.
Boston, Mass. 02115

Seventh Inn Restaurant
67 Providence St.
Boston, MA 02116

New York
Caldron Restaurant
306 East 6th St.
New York, N.Y. 10003

Sou-En Restaurant
2444 Broadway
New York, N.Y. 10024

East West Cookery
105 East 9th St.
New York, N.Y. 10003

Ohio
New World Foodshop
    Restaurant
3408 Telford
Cincinnati, Ohio 45220

CANADA
Vert D-Est Restaurant
969 Rachel St.
Montreal, Canada

*Book Publishers and
Distributors*

Autumn Press
7 Little Rd.
Brookline, MA 02146

Avon Books
959 8th Ave.
New York, N.Y. 10019

Community Health Foun-
    dation
188 Old St.
London, ECI
England

East West Foundation
359 Boylston St.
Boston, MA 02116

East West Journal
233 Harvard St.
Brookline, MA 02146

Erewhon Warehouse
33 Farnsworth St.
Boston, Mass. 02110

G.O.M.F. (George Ohsawa
    Macrobiotic Foundation)
1544 Oak St.
Oroville, Calif. 95965

Happiness Press
160 Wycliff Way
Magalia, Calif. 95954

Red Moon Publications
12 Orpheus St.
London, SE 5
England

Redwing Bookstore
303B Newbury St.
Boston, Mass. 02115

Swan House Publishing Co.
P.O. Box 170
Brooklyn, N.Y. 11223

We personally appreciate those who are spreading the way of life according to the macrobiotic principles throughout North America and the world besides those whose names have appeared in this book. On future occasions more complete reports of the movement will be introduced.

Index